THE
SOCIAL LOGIC
OF
HEALTH

D1121273

THE
SOCIAL LOGIC
OF
HEALTH

Will Wright

Wesleyan University Press
Published by University Press of New England
Hanover and London

To Alexandra and Drew

WESLEYAN UNIVERSITY PRESS
Published by University Press of New England, Hanover, NH 03755
© 1982, 1994 by Will Wright
All rights reserved
Originally published by Rutgers University Press
Printed in the United States of America   5   4   3   2   1
CIP data appear at the end of the book

CONTENTS

PREFACE

Our health care system seems to be in crisis, and there is an ongoing public discussion of how to resolve that crisis. This discussion tends to assume that medicine is doing a good job within its own domain and that the problem is political and economic—that is, a problem of access, profit, rights, regulation. This book argues that the problem is in medicine itself and that the political and economic dilemmas are generated by a fundamental medical misconception about health. Medicine has defined health to be a technical, individual issue when in fact it is a social, institutional issue. This is a conceptual mistake that is partly correct: a large part of health involves the technical repair of individual bodies. But individuals are not simply bodies; they are also social participants, and social institutions are as important as physiology in how bodies work. It is this *social* dimension of individuals, and of individual health, that medicine denies. This conceptual denial, I argue, is generating much of the institutional "crisis" we now face. Indeed, this mistake is generating crises that transcend medicine itself: crises in the environment, in work, in resources, and in political legitimation.

In the realm of health care, there is increasing and effective pressure against the medical definition of health from groups such as women, environmentalists, nutritionists, and naturopaths. All such groups share a sense that health is more of a *social* issue than medicine recognizes. More broadly, issues such as AIDS, violence, and poverty are seen as largely outside the domain of medicine, and yet they are fundamentally issues of health. They are *institutional* issues of health, and medicine has virtually no way to address them.

From this perspective, the current "crisis" is first of all a conceptual issue. We must rethink and clarify our idea of health before we can redesign and reorganize our institutions of health. Without such conceptual investigation, the medical definition of health will remain a sacrosanct assumption, and political and economic strategies will continue to take it for granted. In effect, we will do political and economic tinkering on a confused institutional assumption, easily resulting in more confusion, more bureaucracy, and more waste. The current health dilemmas stem from the assumption that health is strictly physiological, with no social dimension. On this assumption medical costs can only increase, and medical institutions can only become more cumbersome and inefficient. This book challenges that assumption and seeks to redefine health as a *social* concept, so that health care becomes an issue of social theory as well as of individual physiology.

For most of this century scientific medicine has asserted, and generally has been granted, the right to define the concept of health. According to the medical model, the body is essentially a complicated machine, a machine that can be understood and repaired technically. This technical focus on the individual can be contrasted with the more social conception of health of earlier, traditional societies. In these societies health was understood as a moral and social issue, where the physical body functioned in accordance with institutional order. From this perspective an individual could only be healthy within healthy institutions; physical illness was as much a problem of the social order as of the physical body.

The scientific conception of health has stimulated such achievements as sanitation, sterilization, vaccination, and antibiotics, and it has achieved remarkable medical results,

notably the conquest of infectious diseases. It has also, however, created medical and social confusions, and as the twen-
tieth century begins to close these confusions are increasing.
Almost exclusively the medical model has directed health care
toward the constant, competitive development of new medical technology—new drugs, new tests, new machines. Until
recently this technological incentive always appeared as an
incentive for medical hope—a cure for cancer, a preventa-
tive test, a surgical miracle. But now the same technological
focus is also beginning to suggest the possibility of a crisis in
medicine and a failure of health care, primarily because of the
exorbitant expense of the technology.

The current health care crisis is primarily an issue of sky-
rocketing costs, costs that will undermine both medicine and
the economy unless they can be controlled. There are many
viable candidates for the source of this medical inflation: fee-
for-service, malpractice insurance, bureaucratic complexity,
mutual referrals, insurance manipulation, etc. But the best
candidate, the primary source, is almost certainly the constant
pressure for improved, and more expensive, medical technology. Indeed, the development of ever more sophisticated
technology will generally drive all other medical costs, because the doctors, the hospitals, and the patients will always
demand that the available technology be used, in the name
of health, even if the prospects for improved health are small
compared to the potential costs. The increasing expense of
medical technology works on a decreasing margin of health
benefit (primarily the margin of old age), and yet this technology cannot be legitimately resisted or redirected as long as
health is defined as strictly a technical issue of the physiological body (except in cases like living wills, where individuals
choose to resist the "heroic" medical measures of a strictly
technical definition of health.) It is in this sense that scientific
medicine seems to have put itself in something of a histori-

cal, technological bind, particularly in America. Medicine has insisted on defining health as strictly physiological, and the technical expertise associated with that definition has brought medicine great prestige and wealth. But now that same definition is threatening to undermine that prestige, that wealth, and even the basic productivity and stability of our social institutions.

The solution is to redefine the idea of health, for such a new definition, it seems, may soon be imposed politically upon the American medical establishment. The political impetus toward a universal, government-sponsored health plan inevitably involves a more social, less technical definition of health. Any such plan will involve a new idea of what kind of health care for what people is available and appropriate within a more socially defined context. Even if such a plan fails, politically, the social tremors of a new idea of health are already being felt. Such tremors include, for example, the Oregon Health Plan (limiting or "rationing" technological procedures), the medical interventions of Dr. Death (Jack Kevorkian), the payment denials of insurance companies for expensive and marginal technologies, the increasing skepticism toward heroic, technological measures for saving the elderly and the newborn, the growing popularity and legitimacy of "living wills," and the ethical concerns surrounding the new technologies of genetic manipulation.

The technical notion of individual, physiological health is clearly under attack, having in some sense reached its practical, social limit. The idea of health, as opposed to the idea of medicine, is beginning, of necessity, to be understood as having a more contextual, institutional reference. This social idea of health is particularly jarring in America. It is often noted that Americans, more than the citizens of other industrial nations, tend to expect perfect individual health as a right, and thus to expect medicine to live up to its technological, miraculous promise. In other countries, such as England, the people tend to accept the various debilitations of accident and age with more complaisance, thus demonstrating more of a cultural commitment to a *social* idea of health. But in America medicine has had more cultural success with a *technical* idea of health, and so the pressures for a social redefinition will be more disruptive.

In general, scientific medicine has been directed exclusively toward the heroic repair of the individual body, with no suggestion that the idea of health might also imply a measure of institutional criticism and change. In other, more traditional cultures, the idea of health has typically been understood as having a moral and institutional dimension. Primarily, the moral dimension has been directed toward defining both institutional and individual health in terms of the established social tradition. Nevertheless, this alternative concept of health clearly incorporates a social history of the institutional context as well as of the individual body. It is this moral dimension of health that scientific medicine has tried to strip away from the medical idea of health through a strict technical interpretation of the medical model.

Modern society has replaced a reliance on tradition with a reliance on science, and with science has come a social commitment to institutional criticism and change in the name of moral abstractions, such as equality, freedom, and progress. As this new scientific society developed, these moral and social abstractions were carefully detached from any scientific base, so that nothing in scientific nature could have direct social and moral implications. The idea of health, with its obvious reference to empirical nature, could not be construed as a moral term, and so it was identified, by medical science, as a technical term, with no moral, critical content. Scientific society legitimated institutional criticism in the name of justice or freedom, but not in the name of health, because health was

strictly a scientific, physiological term. Throughout this century the institutions of scientific society have been shaped and
buffeted by such moral concerns as freedom and equality, but
not by the moral concerns of health, because health has been
defined as a technical concern of individual bodies. But now
that technical concern is reaching its practical and social limits
as the costs of medical technology begin to undermine both
the credibility of medicine and the stability of the economy.
Inevitably, a more social conception of health will emerge that
inserts a moral and critical dimension within the domain of
medicine.

In this book I argue that the concept of health should be
recognized as a fundamental moral concept, with full-fledged
social and political implications, a concept similar to moral
notions like justice, equality, and freedom. In the medical
context the judgment of ill health always points toward repairing the physiological mechanisms of the body, not toward
repairing the institutional context of the person. For medicine, health is certainly an evaluative term (a good thing) but
only in a technical, mechanical sense, not in a sense that implies legitimate social criticism. If someone is unfree or unequal then their institutions should be critically investigated,
because these judgments are recognized as having moral and
political weight. But if someone is unhealthy, as a medical
judgment, it only suggests that their physiology should be investigated. Individuals can, of course, be responsible for their
own unfreedom or inequality, and so these terms point in both
directions, toward the individual and toward the institutions.
But in particular they point toward the institutional context,
as moral, critical terms. My argument is that the concept of
health also points in both directions, as a full-fledged moral and
social term, with critical institutional implications. Scientific
medicine has systematically denied the institutional implications of the idea of health, through a reliance on the medical

model. But medicine has systematically misunderstood the idea of health, because health necessarily involves the evaluation of social relations as well as the evaluation of the physical body. Our current crisis in health care involves the implications of this scientific mistake, a mistake not only about individuals and their bodies but also about institutions and moral concepts.

Health is not only a full-fledged moral concept, like justice or freedom, it is a special kind of moral concept, with a unique power for social criticism. Judgments of health are always based on, as a necessary foundation, the clear and universal criteria for physiological health. These are the criteria for normal physical functioning, and they involve a straightforward empirical reference, such as broken arms or cracked skulls. The concrete reference for most moral terms—justice, freedom, equality, etc.—can be endlessly debated, since those terms always involve a regress into other moral assumptions with no universal empirical clarity. The institutional implications of justice or freedom change, for example, if individuals are assumed to be competitive rather than communal, or if social order is assumed to be absolutely coercive rather than historically progressive. But it is difficult to debate the moral assumptions involved in a broken arm or a cracked skull or an empty stomach. If health is a moral term, then it must be the fundamental moral term, because all other moral judgments, such as justice or freedom, depend upon an assumption of good health. I argue that health is a moral term, and moreover that it is our most critically potent moral term. If our institutions are judged to be unhealthy, that is, to make people sick, then finally this must be a universal and absolute judgment, a judgment not about cultural values but about empirical human facts.

If health were recognized as a moral term and applied to our modern institutions, it would inevitably have great political impact, particularly on such issues as poverty, the environment, medical care, nutrition, and working conditions. From its technical perspective medicine has systematically denied that the concept of health contains such institutional and moral dimensions, and yet the term inevitably escapes this medical context and begins to imply institutional criticism. For example, we find that automobile exhaust pollutes the air and makes people sick, so the physiological issues of health get caught up in such economic and political issues as global competition, the need for jobs, and government regulation of industry. Indeed, many of our current dilemmas about health care stem from the conceptual necessity of evaluating our institutions in terms of health despite the systematic failure of medicine to do so. In modern America, social criticism tends to be caught in a conceptual dilemma: the legitimate arbiters of health—the doctors and medical professionals—only authorize technical, physiological judgments of health, yet many of our institutions tend to make people sick and thus seem to demand social judgments of health. As a result, the social judgments of health tend to be made by social experts, as opposed to health experts, and so social criticism largely remains a murky issue of moral conundrums (justice, freedom, equality) rather than an objective issue of moral clarity (polluted air, empty stomachs, violent deaths).

The medical establishment is generally unified, with some notable dissension, in its efforts to deny the moral implications of health and to resist any institutional criticism in the name of health. Indeed, from a social perspective the medical effort to capture and neutralize the concept of health, as strictly a physiological concern, becomes as much an issue of institutional legitimation as of effective health care. From the perspective of physiological health the medical model has certainly been effective, and scientific medicine has deserved much of its social and conceptual dominance. But this same conceptual dominance has also protected the status, prestige, and wealth of the medical professionals by removing any professional obligation to engage in social criticism in the name of health. If medicine defined health as a *social* as well as a *technical* term, then the doctors, as medical experts, would also be committed to systematic institutional criticism as well as to physiological repair. That is, the doctors would be committed to criticizing and offending, rather than to serving and joining, the most powerful and successful members of our society.

From a social perspective, the medical profession has clearly protected its own interests by using the medical model to defuse institutional criticism in the name of health. Such criticism, with its obvious empirical reference, would have significant political power, but it would also make the practice of medicine a more contentious and risky endeavor. Scientific medicine has defined health in such a way as to prevent such critical demands, but these demands continue to be felt, by some doctors and many social critics, because the idea of health is inherently social and institutional. Recently, these critical demands have been felt even more strongly because the technological logic of the medical model, with its escalating expense, has begun to undermine both the credibility of medicine and the stability of its institutional base. The social idea of health will always legitimate institutional criticism, even against medicine itself. Now such criticism has begun to undermine medical prestige, while also expanding the legitimate possibilities for health care.

The details of the argument are in the text, and among those details is a critique of the philosophical distinction between facts and values. According to this distinction facts cannot entail values, which means that value judgments can only be derived from other value judgments, not from empirical facts. Discussion of such things as justice and freedom, then, will always remain in the realm of values and cannot be connected with the realm of facts. I argue, however, that the concept of health bridges the fact-value gap in a decisive way, because the judgment of health (a good thing) necessarily connects physiological facts (healthy lungs) with institutional values (industrial pollution). Health necessarily involves both physiological and institutional dimensions; as a result, institutional values can be logically derived from physiological facts, because physiological facts are necessarily laden with fundamental human and social values. If properly analyzed, the idea of health disrupts our standard conceptual assumptions about moral concepts. These standard assumptions define a natural world that is empirical, objective, and neutral—a natural world with no inherent moral dimensions. This is the world of science, including medical science; my social analysis of health can be seen as an effort to disrupt this world and to argue that necessary institutional values and criticism can be derived from the empirical, physiological facts of human health.

My argument suggests that modern institutions will come under increasing social criticism in the name of health, despite the best efforts of medicine to neutralize the concept. Such institutional criticisms were already apparent when I wrote the book, and they have been gaining force and legitimacy since then. Perhaps the most severe and effective criticism has been directed toward the medical institutions themselves and their legal and technical hegemony over health. In the last ten years scientific medicine has significantly expanded its tolerance for and openness to broader conceptions of human health. Under pressure from women, nutritionists, chiropractors, and others, some doctors have begun to think that health may be more than strictly a technical issue of physiological repair.

The women's health movement has consistently attacked the medical establishment in the name of health, arguing that what medicine implicitly understood as health was male health, as represented by the male body. In response, the National Institutes of Health have recently begun to expand research on women's health, in effect recognizing women's issues as a valid medical concern. This medical recognition has been politically motivated, from external pressure, rather than medically motivated. Further, hospitals and doctors have begun to change their medical attitudes toward childbirth, also under external pressure from women, so that now there is increased use of birthing centers and of nurse-midwives. In essence, medicine is at least beginning to think of childbirth as less of a disease and as more a part of normal life, that is, as something to be done in a comfortable, home-like setting, with medical support available but not intrusive. Also, issues of breast cancer have become more of a central focus for medicine, largely as a result of organized attention from women's groups.

Another recent, and rather successful, source of external pressure on medicine, in the name of health, has come from alternative conceptions of medicine, conceptions such as acupuncture, chiropractic, homeopathy, nutrition, naturopathy, and Ayurvedic. The American medical establishment is slowly and sporadically beginning to relax its historic, rabid resistance to such alternative strategies, largely as a result of increasing public interest in these strategies and decreasing satisfaction with scientific medicine. Medical resistance is still intense, but the signs of grudging tolerance and acceptance are apparent. Most striking, perhaps, has been the recent creation of the Office of Alternative Medicine at the National Institutes of Health, where small amounts of money, along with governmental legitimacy, will be given to support research into alternative medical procedures. In the realm of health insurance, alternative strategies seem to be gaining some credibility, although resistance is still significant. A majority of the insurers, for example, now cover acupuncture treatments, and many companies are beginning to cover nutritional approaches to such issues as heart disease. In other areas, the American

Medical Association reversed a long-standing policy and announced in 1992 that it was ethical for doctors to refer patients to chiropractors. The number of homeopathic practitioners has been rapidly increasing since the seventies, and some homeopathic remedies are now being advertised on television. The mind-body conception of Ayurvedic, an ancient Indian approach to health, has been gaining both patients and medical study. Bill Moyers's book, *The Healing Mind*, spent many weeks on the best-seller lists. An increasing number of medical schools, including Harvard and Georgetown, are beginning to offer courses in alternative and unorthodox medicine. In the last ten years a broader, more open conception of health has greatly increased its power to pressure, disrupt, and expand the narrow focus of the medical model.

In a broader context the issues of health are legitimating an increasing criticism of economic and political institutions, particularly from an environmental perspective. Environmental problems are becoming more global and intractable, and as such are becoming more politically prominent. Broadly, these environmental problems can be divided into two basic categories: the loss of wilderness and the loss of health. The first has to do generally with soiling our own nest, that is, with losing, perhaps forever, the wild places and the natural rhythms that have always enveloped human life. The second category involves the ways in which pollution and degradation make people sick. Over the last decade or so this second category of problems has begun to have the greatest political impact, because these health problems generate the most immediate, powerful, and convincing institutional criticisms. Dilemmas such as the greenhouse effect, ozone depletion, the loss of biodiversity, and the loss of agriculture are now being seen as primarily issues of health, and from this perspective more political muscle is being exercised and more solutions offered.

According to a United Nations report released in 1992, global malnutrition and skin cancer are increasing, as well as water and farmland degradation, while at least one billion people breathe unhealthy air. As a response, the U.N. and the World Bank have begun to organize conferences on sustainability and environmental concerns. The World Bank has admitted its past environmental inattention and has begun to assess the environmental impacts of its developmental projects in poorer countries. The Earth Summit in Rio has focused world attention on the interrelations between pollution, denudation, poverty, and health. In this context, international agreements have been negotiated to protect the ozone layer, to reduce the greenhouse effect, and to protect biodiversity. This last agreement, called the Convention on Biological Diversity, is particularly interesting. Signed by 167 nations, including the United States, it is directed toward the protection of plants, animals, and microorganisms across the globe. But the political legitimation of the treaty is not the radical environmental ethic of ecocentrism, where no species (i.e., humans) is seen as privileged and all species are understood as having an equal right to live and flourish. Rather, the treaty is legitimated by an economic incentive, where the protection of wilderness would generate economic development in the field of health care. The treaty idea is that both rich and poor nations would share in the profits of biotechnology, that is, the profits from the new medical products and improved crops resulting from the industrial and scientific exploration of genetic diversity. Diversity is being given political protection because of its potential for health care, not because of its inherent value as wilderness. In effect, environmental attention in the form of institutional criticism is increasing, primarily through a focus on health, where health is understood as a social, global, and environmental, as well as a medical, concern.

Over the last decade the idea of health has increasingly

organized effective political attacks on scientific medicine (as
narrow and technical) as well as on industrial production (as
ecologically indifferent). The important conceptual point is
that the notion of health can always be mobilized for social and
political goals, despite the quiescence of medicine. But the
political point is that these attacks have not helped much. Despite the effective moral expansion of the idea of health, medicine is still becoming more technical and detached and the
environment is still getting worse. The fundamental conceptual point is that institutional criticism in the name of health
must become far more powerful and effective. The idea of economic health, for example, must begin to be understood as an
issue of *health* as well as an issue of economics. Currently, we
think of economic health as involving such issues as productivity, competition, and quality, not such issues as violence,
hunger, pollution, depression, and fear. Scientific medicine
has successfully separated the idea of health from the evaluation of our institutions, which often means that a healthy economy must make many people sick. Our idea of health must be
expanded, as a moral concept, and our doctors must become
more critical. But primarily we must begin to reconceptualize
our institutions and their moral legitimation. We must begin
to think more carefully about such things as justice and freedom and equality. When people can be politically free while
constantly hungry, polluted, fearful, and sick, then there must
be some conceptual flaw in the way we understand our institutions, our lives, and our health.

Two of the most visible health problems in contemporary
America are AIDS and violence. At the social level AIDS involves sexual promiscuity and drug use, and violence involves
the loss of jobs, the breakdown of the family, and the drug
trade. These are clearly institutional concerns, but they are
also health issues, and they should be understood as residing
in the conceptual domain of health. Medicine searches for vac-

cines and cures, but often it is the social order, not germs, that
makes people sick. Even if a vaccine for AIDS could be found,
there will be no vaccine for violence other than productive
jobs, enforceable laws, and stable lives. If these institutional
issues were recognized as problems of health, and thus as part
of the legitimate domain of our health professionals, then the
doctors could use their political clout to criticize our institutions as easily as they use it to maximize their income.

Our most obvious and pervasive health problem is poverty,
or rather the myriad problems of physical and mental health
that result from widespread and systemic poverty. Poverty is
known to be our leading cause of poor health, and yet it is not
discussed, politically or medically, as an issue of health. The
health effects of poverty are discussed in the text, accompanied
by certain data on poverty, and while this data could be slightly
updated, the basic point about poverty and health remains the
same. Indeed, both the numbers of the poor and the numbers
of the sick and injured among the poor have increased in the
last decade, primarily because of the loss of jobs. Similarly, the
relative position of the United States with respect to international comparisons on health indices has changed minimally,
if at all, in the last ten years. When George Schieber and
his colleagues investigated twenty-four countries in 1991, they
concluded: "In comparison with other major industrial countries, health care in the United States costs more per person
and per unit of service, is less accessible to a large portion of its
citizens, is provided at a more intensive level, and offers com-
paratively poor gross outcomes."[1] Medicine in America is less
effective than it should be, according to international comparisons, and part of the reason is that America accepts a greater
degree of poverty as institutionally legitimate. American medicine still does not recognize poverty as an issue of health, and
so while the statistics in the text may have changed slightly,
the conceptual and social points remain exactly the same.

As our medical and institutional crises grow, and our technology expands, the idea of health becomes more complicated and confusing. Primarily, this is an issue of physical health, as I have suggested, but it is also an issue of mental health, particularly with respect to a recent medical possibility for the mind. This new possibility is offered by the mood-altering drug Prozac (and its cognates), a drug that seems not only to relieve depression and anger, but also to make people better, in the sense of wittier, more confident, more sexual, more energetic, etc. Apparently, the drug has minimal negative side effects, compared to its positive effects, and so it raises the interesting issue of whether health is even a natural state anymore. Is good health something people have when their bodies and their society are functioning well, or will it become something that can only be achieved artificially, through chemical enhancement? Will good health become something that is defined by chemical access, and is this the next implication of a scientific and technical definition of health? So far the drugs offering this kind of improvement have tended to become illegal, presumably because of their negative health consequences. But when some such drug as Prozac finally does improve us without ill effects, the idea of health, among other things, will take another confusing conceptual turn.

In the text I argue that institutions that make people systematically and unnecessarily sick cannot be considered healthy institutions, despite the collective but separated wisdoms of social theory and medical science. The image of what *could* be considered healthy institutions was probably clearer to me a decade ago than it is now, but the necessity of investigating our institutions with more coherent concepts is even more clear now. Perhaps in the last ten years we have all become more cynical about institutions as socialism has collapsed, the environment may be collapsing, our cities seem to be collapsing, and the global economy has created massive distortions of health, work, poverty, and war. Amidst all of this we still tend to think of our institutions, whether in economics, politics, or social theory, as though they were independent of issues of health. We tend to think about our institutions, conceptually, as though they were derived from some Revealed Truth about human nature, rather than as though they should be designed to make our lives possible and our societies sustainable.

In the new context of the global economy, the idea of *sustainability* is probably the key. The idea of sustainability is like the idea of health, in the sense that both are somewhat vague, both have moral power, and both provide a constant critical reference against the asserted moral authority of established institutions. In essence, the idea of sustainability is simply a generalization of the social level of the idea of health, since good health implies the maximum possible sustainability of an individual life. This means that we must begin to criticize and reorganize our institutions in the name of sustainability, as the social and ecological equivalent of institutional health. On our small planet, with its failing environment, we must begin to be more careful about our social and moral concepts and about the institutions they endorse. The technical concepts of science have brought us enormous benefits and have generally legitimated our modern institutions. But these scientific concepts entail serious social incoherencies, which have now started to become institutional, technological, and environmental disasters. Within the domain of science itself, as I have argued in another place,[2] we must begin to rethink our idea of physical nature, so that our technology and our institutions become conceptually committed to the idea of sustainability. And within the domain of medical science we must begin to rethink our idea of health, so that medicine becomes an issue of social criticism as well as physiological repair. The idea of health must be recognized as a unique and fundamental moral concept, and if it is then we will begin to look at our bodies, our institutions, and our concepts differently.

NOTES

1. George Schieber et al., "Health Care Systems in Twenty-four Countries," *Health Affairs* (fall 1991), p. 23.
2. Will Wright, *Wild Knowledge: Science, Language, and Social Life in a Fragile Environment* (Minneapolis: University of Minnesota Press, 1993).

THE CONCEPT
OF HEALTH

Health is a topic of constant concern these days, from the issue of national insurance to the research on cancer, from the image of the doctor as savior to the proliferation of books on vitamins, nutrition, self-healing, and holistic medicine. Yet in all this discussion the question of just exactly what health is, of what it means to be healthy, is seldom raised. The issues of care availability, financing, research, environment, and education are typically addressed as though the definition of health is somehow naturally understood by everyone. I propose to challenge this assumption by looking closely at the idea of health, at what we mean when we say that someone or something is healthy. In particular, I intend to use this investigation to question whether the idea of human health that is implicitly contained in our basic institutions of health care can possibly be adequate, or even sensible.

In order to explore this topic in this way I shall undertake an extended analysis of the concept of health, of how it is used to account for, justify, and motivate actions and decisions. All discussions of medical structures must necessarily be confused and incomplete until the issue of just exactly what it is we are looking for with our health-related institutions and research has been more clearly and systematically understood. There is, of course, a hidden argument in this assertion, and it is this methodological assumption that I wish to make explicit and defend briefly in this introduction.

My underlying argument is that if we are ever to understand the institutions and activities of our social life, we must
in some fundamentally prior sense understand the concepts
we use to organize, structure, and justify that life. That is,
we must make rigorous conceptual analysis the first step of
social analysis. Indeed, this work is as much an effort to
demonstrate the practical, institutional importance of analyzing the concepts we use as it is an effort to clarify the notion,
and thus the ongoing discussions, of health. Generally, today
only philosophers are exposed to systematic training in conceptual analysis, and this training has become so formalized
that it is virtually devoid of any discussion or investigation of
social context. On the other hand, sociologists, economists,
and political scientists learn how to investigate social context
through sophisticated data-gathering techniques, yet these
techniques include virtually no critical consciousness directed toward the concepts they incorporate. An extended
and valuable literature addresses the question of whether
"objective" data are possible in the social sciences, given the
need to rely on everyday, socially relevant concepts in research, but this discussion is not concerned with conceptual
analysis as a research tool for social understanding. Rather, it
is oriented toward mitigating the assumed bias involved in
using everyday meanings in "objective" research. In other
words, the concepts themselves become objects of study according to standard social scientific techniques for raising
questions and obtaining information.

But the basic issues are: How are the questions raised?
What questions need to be asked? If a fundamentally confused or ambiguous concept underlies the recognition that
there is a problem to be solved, that more information is
needed, then the answers obtained, the information gath-
ered, will be confused and ambiguous no matter how sophisticated and "objective" the techniques employed. That is, if

the "health" that physicians understand as the goal of their profession is in some way conceptually different from the "health" that insurance companies finance or the "health" that environmentalists feel is threatened or that holistic practitioners feel is achievable, then the arguments and evidence that each group advances or that social scientists advance in support of different positions will be essentially incommensurable and thus useless as the basis for intelligent institutional decisions. Without conceptual elucidation, the discussions of health care, however elaborate and sophisticated, may fail to be socially applicable, if indeed such is their intention.

Another such concept is the notion of intelligence, a concept that is used to motivate and justify many educational and promotional decisions in our society; indeed, the notion of education itself is such a concept. We can all support the usefulness of the idea of intelligence, just as we can all agree on the need for education, but do intelligence tests or grading systems really measure what it is we think we are supporting, and do educational institutions really provide what it is we think we need? If we are trying to improve our educational system, or use intelligence, or maximize health, then we must know what it is we are trying to improve, or use, or maximize. We must systematically elucidate and articulate clear and acceptable references for terms like health and intelligence before we can usefully investigate the social context for the purpose of maximizing their occurrence.

The concepts of health and intelligence, together with such terms as justice, freedom, peace, and progress, all share a deep and revealing ambiguity in the common usage. We desire all of them, we create institutions to produce or encourage them, and we are never quite sure that what those institutions provide is indeed what we wanted to obtain. Justice, for example, is something we all support and seek, and we have created an elaborate system of justice—laws, courts, police, lawyers—in order to achieve it. But with respect to any specific action or decision of this system, any one of us might argue that what was achieved was not justice but injustice or a miscarriage of justice. That is, we have established an institutional arrangement that by definition dispenses justice: justice has been done, justice has prevailed, and so forth. On the other hand, we are also aware that the justice that has prevailed may not be justice at all: the wrong man may have been convicted, the poor have generally less access to legal protection than the rich, presidents can defy the Constitution with impunity. Clearly, at least two notions of justice are at work here, and this simple ambiguity has had, and continues to have, significant ramifications for our institutions and our social order.

At the conceptual level, this ambiguity means, among other things, that our system of justice has been established, or at least we believe it has been established, in order to achieve a systematic rendering of justice of a type we somehow understand intuitively or naturally—that is, a concept of justice understood independently of the system of justice itself. We do not understand the concept of justice to mean that which is dispensed by the legal institutions; rather we use our understanding of the concept of justice to evaluate and critique the decisions handed down by those institutions. Now, where does this understanding come from? Where do we get the sense, which all of us experience from time to time, that in a particular instance justice has miscarried, even though all of the formal procedures of justice have worked properly? Further, is there one more or less universal standard sense of justice that everyone shares in some tacit, unreflective way, or does each person appeal to his or her own more or less private, individual sense of justice, which may or may not have much in common with another person's sense? In the first case, the validity of the institutions of justice would be measured against their normal ability to approximate this universal sense; in the second case, it would be measured against their success in achieving an acceptable compromise among divergent senses. In any case, the importance of the conceptual analysis becomes clear: we must understand how a concept like justice functions in a social order if we are to construct legitimate institutions supporting that concept.

The same argument applies to the concept of health: there must be a coherent meaning to the judgment of health that is not determined by the medical institutions we have constructed for the achievement of health. Rather this meaning, whether individual or social, must be understood inherently in some way and thus be available for the evaluation of the success of those institutions. My central concern is to analyze this meaning and to explore what that analysis implies about our health, the medical establishment, and our social order. In the case of health—and this will be a central point of the analysis—the judgments we naturally make, particularly concerning our own health, must be at least to some degree uniform, since none of us would think ourselves or anyone else healthy while suffering from a broken arm, or cancer, or a bullet in the stomach. Thus it is possible to claim that our understanding of the concept of health rests significantly on some reasonably straightforward and universal meanings in a way that it is not possible, at least on the face of it, to make a similar claim about such concepts as justice, freedom, or progress, where the meanings seem to be much more dependent upon individual or cultural values. This implies that health is a unique concept, and this uniqueness will not only serve to illuminate some of the relations between the physical and the social in our society but will also help us to understand how concepts work in our lives.

I would like to take note of one other property of concepts before turning to the analysis itself. Most of us, if we were not philosophers and if we were pressed about what concepts are, would say something to the effect that they stand for *things*, particularly those concepts that refer to material objects. That is, the concept of tree stands for the object "the tree" out in the yard, or the concept of car stands for the object "the car" out on the street, and so forth. But even with respect to our own ordinary understanding, this is not strictly the case, as is easy to see from thinking about a situation where you might ask to borrow a friend's car, and the friend replies, "Sure, but you can't have the keys," or the case where you are about to be attacked by a crazed grizzly and you ask John nearby if he has a gun, and he says yes, and you begin to feel better, and then find out that he has no bullets. In other words, if you ask to borrow a car or a gun, you are not just asking to borrow the material object; you are asking for the use of its function, its active or dynamic properties. Few of us, in a life-threatening situation, would ask to borrow both a gun and bullets, but if someone offered us a gun we could use and then we discovered that there were no bullets, we would think of that as odd—we might even think the person had lied to us, or worse. Thus we include in the meaning of the term "gun" not just the metal object, but the fact that it will shoot, just as we include in the meaning of the term "car" the fact that it will run. The point is that virtually every concept we use normally in dealing with daily life refers not only to a thing but also to a function, to a set of relationships with other things, to the accomplishment or potential accomplishment of associated events. We would not call an object that looked like a screwdriver a screwdriver if it did not screw screws, for example. Concepts have meaning not as names for things but through participation in an elaborate network of associated meanings and implied relationships.

Once again, few of us would buy or borrow a gun in order to shoot game or protect our lives without also making sure we had some bullets. And if we told others that we had a gun, we may not mention bullets, but they would almost certainly understand that we had them. But suppose we lived in a society in which guns had just been introduced, so that their abilities were commonly known but not their workings. Suppose, then, that we wanted a gun and that some unscrupulous or ignorant person gave us one—that is, gave us the metal object—but failed to tell us about or give us any bullets. Then, in the only sense that matters, we did not get a gun, and under certain circumstances the results could be quite disastrous. Because we were familiar with the concept but failed truly to understand it and its necessary relationship with other things and events, we were sold or given something that seemed to be what we wanted but in fact was not, something that, moreover, could turn out to be seriously detrimental.

In the following chapters I suggest that something like this may be happening in this country with respect to the concept and the institutions of health. We may be spending a lot of effort and money to get something we have all heard about and want but do not fully understand; therefore, the real object may in some important way be contradictory to what we are obtaining. What we tend to buy when we go to a doctor or a hospital is the repairing of our physical body. But, like other concepts, health is meaningful only in terms of a set of social relationships, and it may be that the medical establishment is selling us the gun without the bullets— giving us the appearance of health while at the same time participating actively in the structuring of our relationships so as to inhibit, and perhaps even undermine, the occurrence of health. This possibility arises through the recognition that concepts such as health become meaningful only through their interdependence with other concepts and events. It is this interdependence, the ways in which the idea of health is integrated into our ideas of valuable and rewarding social relationships, that must be explored if we are to understand fully the implications of the issues of health for social life.

CHAPTER ONE

THE HEALTH
OF HUMANS

What does it mean to be healthy? In particular, what does it mean for human beings to be healthy? This latter qualification makes it a complicated and sometimes confusing issue. Although only one judgment, one set of criteria, is really relevant in deciding the health of a plant or an animal, in the case of a human being two such judgments are inevitably (with rare exceptions) crucial in any final evaluation of health, and thus the possibility exists that two distinct, even contradictory, sets of criteria will be invoked. In the case of an apparently ailing dog or rose bush, we either make or call for an expert opinion as to what curative action would be appropriate and then proceed on that basis. Even if we called for two or a dozen expert opinions, it would only be to test the competence of a particular expert, since presumably the criteria used by any one for the evaluation of plant or animal health—that is, the biological-chemical model of organic functioning—would be the same as that used by all the others. (Unless, of course, an expert were consulted who might prescribe conversation or classical music for the rose bush or alpha waves or pyramids for the dog, a not negligible possibility in some parts of Los Angeles.)

In the case of a human being, however, the procedure is necessarily more complex. When hurt or ill, we will most naturally consult a doctor and generally follow his or her advice. But as a part of the doctor's determination and recommendation, he or she will generally, whenever possible, consult with the patient as to the history, symptoms, effects, and often even the treatment of the illness. That is, the response to human illness and suffering almost invariably involves some degree of negotiation between an "expert's" knowledge of proper biological and physiological functioning and an individual's idea of how it feels to be healthy, how it feels to be ill, and what kinds of procedures and treatments are compatible with the former. For example, many patients will refuse, against all medical advice, certain surgical procedures (such as amputation), certain drugs, and certain kinds of treatment (such as radiation) because they feel that the suffering involved is not compatible with their idea of health. On the other hand, many patients will, again in defiance of medical expertise, undertake various forms of treatment, from vitamin C to laetrile, from chiropractic to the laying on of hands, because they believe such treatment to be compatible with and beneficial to their own idea of health.

This is not to say that these latter procedures are in fact truly curative and that the doctors are wrong, just as it is not to say that the former medical procedures are in fact truly debilitating and that once again the doctors are wrong. Rather, these examples indicate significant divergences over questions of health and how to achieve it among human beings. A more obvious example is the common feeling that the doctors have in some way "screwed up" with respect to our own health or that of a friend—and not only in the sense that an individual doctor made a medical mistake, as exemplified by the rising incidence of malpractice cases, but in the more general sense that doctors cannot be expected to be responsive to a real human situation, to the concrete needs, fears, and suffering of a particular individual. Both in word-of-mouth folk wisdom and in an increasing number of reports from researchers and critics, including many doctors,

it is being suggested that in most cases we are better off to
avoid doctors, and especially hospitals, if we possibly can.
Clearly two very different criteria of health are being invoked: the medical-physiological idea on the one hand and
the unarticulated but generally shared and communicable
experience of our own health on the other. The problem,
then, is this: whereas the doctors are experts with respect to
health in general, every person is in some sense an expert
with respect to his or her own health in a way that dogs and
rose bushes are not experts with respect to their own health,
since they cannot give advice, evaluate procedures, or refuse
certain treatments.

The inevitability of two experts in any particular case—
one with great technical sophistication but limited personal
understanding and the other with abundant personal sensi-
tivity but generally limited technical comprehension and access—is the complicating factor in any discussion and analysis of human health. It would not be so great a problem if
we could be sure that these two experts, coming from necessarily different perspectives, shared the same basic criteria
with respect to the evaluation of an individual's health. Many
observers have argued that this is indeed the case with respect to modern medicine, and in fact, the legitimation of
the medical profession rests upon this assumption. Doctors
are seen as having the true conception and understanding of
health, and although the rest of us may have an intuitive and
often medically helpful sense of when we have it and when
we do not, with respect to the explanation, evaluation, and
treatment of ill health, we must, for all practical purposes,
give ourselves over to the superior knowledge of the doctors,
more or less as though we are dogs or rose bushes. All of
us may have some competence in recognizing our own ill
health, but when it comes to explaining and treating health
breakdowns, anyone who is not an M.D. or does not rely on

the bio-physiological model of medical science can only be lucky or wrong, for human health is exactly and only what this model defines it to be. Since this is what health is objectively, either we all share the same conception of it, and thus the same criteria for evaluating it—in which case our limited expertise with respect to our own health pales into insignificance before the far more refined and sophisticated expertise of the doctors—or those of us who have a different conception, and thus different criteria, are either simply confused and mistaken or are charlatans. This is the standard medical view of health as we have it today, and most of us have little option in most practical situations but to surrender to this dominant conception, though in our anger and frustration we·still manage to cling to the sense that our own health at least is a somewhat more complex matter than this.

I do not believe that this difference between the human experience of health and the doctors' bio-physiological conception of it can be resolved quite as easily as the doctors suggest. The basic dilemma seems to be whether health is a concept that can be defined objectively and technically by medical scientists or whether it is a concept that refers finally and decisively to a quality of human experience that cannot be reduced to physiological processes. If the former is the case, the doctors are indeed the true experts regarding health, and we must adjust our understanding and trust to become ever more compatible with their objective diagnoses. If the latter is the case, then there are indeed, at least at present, two necessarily divergent and almost inevitably conflicting criteria for the evaluation of human health: one that rests solely upon a model of organic life as such, surely an important consideration for human beings, and one that depends much more intimately upon the nature and experience of *human* life as opposed to other forms of organic functioning, surely also an important consideration for human beings.

I shall argue that the latter is indeed the case and that the medical model cannot be an adequate conceptualization of the dimensions of human health. That such a discrepancy exists and that it ill serves the interests of patients has been remarked upon by many doctors themselves. For example, Dr. George L. Engel, professor of medicine and psychiatry at the University of Rochester School of Medicine, notes:

> Patients are the ones who tell us that doctors do not communicate well, that they do not really listen, that they seem insensitive to personal needs and individual differences, that they often neglect the person in their zeal to pursue diagnostic and treatment procedures. . . . These complaints, and others, bespeak the public's awareness of grave deficiencies in the medical establishment's knowledge of and ability to handle rationally the human experience of being ill.
>
> A primary contributor to this gap between the medical profession and the public it is meant to serve is the fundamental difference between the patient's criteria for health and well-being and those of the physician, a difference which exists even though culturally and intellectually both patient and physician share a cultural inheritance which includes the biomedical model of disease. For the patient, the ultimate criteria are psychosocial, even when the complaint is physical. Patient's criteria have to do with how one feels, how one functions, how one relates with others; with the ability to love, to work, to struggle, to seek options and make choices. The physician, in contrast, while ostensibly attentive to such concerns, nonetheless is wont to consider such criteria as "merely subjective." For the physician, the real criteria for status and outcome of health

and disease are physical measures, for whose determination increasingly elegant and sensitive instruments
are available. (Engel, p. 261)

To argue successfully that two incompatible sets of criteria
exist for understanding and using the concept of health, I
must address two distinct questions. First, why should anyone believe that this second set of criteria, the one that
refers to the unique experiences of human life, not only
exists but is also relevant, since all of our medical wisdom
seems to deny it? It is one thing to assert its significance, as
Engel does and as I have to this point, but it is another thing
to argue in the face of the obvious achievements of medical
science that these criteria remain valuable, and even primary, in any understanding of human health. Second, what
are the critical differences between the two sets of criteria?
In particular, since the medical criteria are apparently well-
established, I must indicate with some precision what constitutes this second set of criteria, that is, what it means to
be a healthy human being as opposed to being a healthy dog
or a healthy rose bush. The answer to this second question,
with various digressions and elaborations, will compose the
body of this book. In the remainder of this chapter, I shall
suggest a conceptual answer to the first question.

My argument about the necessary reference of the concept of health as it is applied to human beings depends upon
a more general analysis of how concepts work in our lives.
One characteristically human activity is to use a language,
that is, to relate to the world conceptually. In any particular
society at any given time in history the people of that society
have available to them a conceptual system, a deeply layered
and overlapping framework of concepts that moves from the
very particular to the very general and with which they cover
and understand the elements of their experience. These con-

cepts mutually refer and interrelate in such a way as to generate explanations that allow the people of the society to make sense of their lives, to act on the world in such a way that the expected and desired results of those actions are generally obtained. In order for this to be true across different societies, given the basic uniformity of the natural environment—seasons come and go regularly, rocks are not edible, avalanches kill people—it must be the case that the explanations and the conceptual structures, though they vary widely, from science to mysticism, all to some degree rest on a set of essentially similar concepts that reflect and point to important and uniform differences among things in the natural world. That is, all human societies must employ concepts that distinguish with functional precision between rocks and animals, trees and birds, land and water, plants and soil. Without such distinctions the members of a society might try to walk on water and swim on land or, more significantly, in time of famine they might try to stalk, kill, and eat a rock. But of course such things are not possible, and the reason they are not possible is that making such distinctions is concomitant with being a human being, that is, with using a language, with belonging to a society, and with understanding the world in such a way that it is possible to act on it successfully with respect to survival. To beings that relate to the world conceptually, such basic distinctions—however these concepts may then be interrelated by explanatory metaphysics and ideology—are an integral part of existence.

And of course rocks are not just distinguished from animals, they are distinguished from all things that are not rocks. As Saussure and others have pointed out, concepts get their meaning not from what they are but from what they are not. To be meaningful the concept of "rock" must imply a set of criteria that allows its users to understand the crucial aspects of being a rock, aspects that prevent whatever satis-

fies those criteria from being anything except a rock. Each
particular thing has distinctive characteristics that are more
or less unambiguously shared by other members of the same
group but not by things outside that group. It is the business
of a concept to capture and point to those distinctive characteristics, and it is the business of a conceptual framework to
make enough of these conceptual distinctions so that no important—that is, survival-connected—differences are systematically confused or ambiguous.

One of the conceptual distinctions important for any society, is the difference between being a human being and
being something else, say a rock or a tree or an animal or a
building. Clearly this is an important distinction, for in a
society where it was not made precisely, the people might
mistake an advancing army for a herd of elephants or someone might try to bring a building home for dinner. More
seriously, it is clear that human beings can interact with one
another in ways they cannot interact with rocks or buildings
or animals and that this difference must be articulated in the
language. The telling difference will be between humans and
animals, since humans share many, if not most, of their major characteristics with animals. But as is clear to all of us,
and as the conceptual distinction implies, humans are cru-
cially different from animals. In particular, we can communicate conceptually with humans in a way we cannot with
animals. This is why, for example, human slaves, so long as
they do not revolt, make far better workers—they can be
given contingent instructions, they can be held responsible
—than do animals, no matter how well trained. These distinguishing characteristics, even though they cannot easily
be theoretically articulated, are necessarily contained within
the concept of human being, and we all understand them
naturally. That is, all languages make this conceptual distinction, and all users of those languages understand implicitly

in virtually all cases of practical significance how to use those concepts properly. In almost every case we all know in some natural and reasonably unambiguous way how to distinguish between human beings and other things, and this knowledge entails that we all understand naturally, inherent in our use of the language, a set of critical criteria for recognizing what it means to be human. This does not mean, of course, that we always treat other people equally as human beings; indeed, I am making no claim about the myriad ideological possibilities of distinguishing between groups of human beings in terms of quality and worth. What I am suggesting is that, no matter how badly a society may treat a particular group or class of humans, even if this group is systematically referred to as subhuman or as animals, the people of the society are still never conceptually confused in any practical situation about whether those people are in fact humans or animals. Indeed, as was systematically demonstrated in the German concentration camps, the specifically human need of individuals for conceptual coherence in their lives creates the possibility of far more intense cruelty and mistreatment toward people than could ever be the case toward animals.

We have established that the linguistically necessary concept of being human entails at least an implicit understanding of what it uniquely and practically means to be human. Yet the business of being human involves many different aspects. In particular it involves certain physical characteristics, as does being a rock or a tree or an animal, as well as specific types of activities. Most of the physical characteristics associated with being human, apart from such things as the size of the brain and the opposing thumb, are similar to the physical characteristics of certain species of animals. Moreover, many of the characteristic activities of human life, such as eating, sexual intercourse, and collecting in interdependent groups, are also shared by some animal species.

Some human activities, however, are not shared by any types of animals, and it is here, it would seem, that we can most likely identify the distinguishing characteristics of being human: for example, using language to conceptualize and explain the world, taking action based on conceptual understanding, using concepts to envision alternative possibilities and thus make choices, being both able and required to communicate conceptually, and taking responsibility for our choices and thus for our actions, that is, being able to produce ourselves out of our own efforts, our labor. These kinds of characteristics seem to be good candidates for the uniquely human activities, but whatever they are, it is clear that such distinguishing activities do exist and that they must in large degree be processes, the exhibiting of particular types of possibilities through interaction and communication. In other words, human beings are human beings not primarily because they *have* certain things but because they are able to *do* certain things that other animals cannot.

This discussion, of course, rests upon the idea of being human under optimum conditions; that is, it is intended to suggest that there is a norm of being human, an abstraction that characterizes the most general and normal experience of human life. Such a norm, I have argued, must inhere in the concept of being human if we are to use that concept meaningfully and successfully. And when we do use it meaningfully and successfully, we almost always use it with respect to real people in everyday, concrete situations: even the decision to talk to someone, to drive down the street, to sit in a crowded theater involves the tacit recognition that the other person, the other drivers, the other members of the audience are normal human beings. But real people do not always exist under optimum conditions. Since being human does not depend upon whether one has something or not but rather on whether one can do something or not, there must obviously be varying degrees to which a real person can be recognized as meeting the norm of human activity. People are more or less fragile and temporal, and there will always be at any particular time some number of them who at that time could not meet all the criteria inherent in the concept of being human. It follows, then, that either such people can no longer be considered human, which is nonsense, or that there must be some way for them to be understood as still human but as relieved, for a time, of some of the expectations of activity that that designation normally carries (compare Parsons's concept of the sick role [1964, chap. 10]). In other words, since the distinguishing characteristics of being human are certain kinds of activities, there must be a concept naturally available in the language that indicates the condition under which an individual can be expected to fulfill those activities, and there must be another concept, or a series of concepts, that indicates the gradations of conditions under which an individual would be understood as not being able to engage fully in those activities. It is my contention that the former concept must of necessity be the concept of health and that the latter concepts are those of ill health, sickness, disease, injury, and the like.

Health, I believe, when it is applied to human beings, is the concept in the natural language that characterizes the state in which individuals can be and are fully human. Such a concept must exist because it makes one of those important distinctions that exist in the natural world, the distinction between an individual being fully or less than fully conscious, active, and accountable, a distinction that is crucial, for example, for the determination of guilt in our legal system. It is a distinction that involves an optimum condition, and health certainly refers to an optimum condition, one that all of us seek and desire. Since such a concept must exist, the only real issue becomes whether health is that concept, or whether we must look elsewhere for it. When the question is put in this way, it is clear that there is nowhere else to look, that health is the only possibility and that it plays exactly that role in our normal usage of language and in our natural understanding of what it means for a human being to be healthy. The only occasion for doubt would be the overwhelming strength of the doctors' assertion that health refers to a technical and objective condition of physiological processes, not to the definitive characteristics of the essence of human life.

The judgment of health, then, as it is used normally by nonprofessionals, entails a prior understanding of what it means for a person to be able, more or less, to interact according to his or her full capabilities as a human being. This understanding is not of the scholarly or theoretical sort but is rather a sense, a knowledge, integral to the use of the concept; indeed, the understanding constitutes the concept. This knowledge, I have argued, is necessarily present wherever the concept is used, and the concept is necessarily used in all human societies. Thus in a society like ours, where the concept is also made the subject of a detailed scholarly and theoretical analysis and where analysis conflicts in some important ways with the natural use and understanding of the term, it is clear that at least two sets of criteria are available for understanding and evaluating what it means to be healthy, one explicit and articulate and the other intuitive and inherent. It is incumbent upon any analyst of the concept of health to try to make this second set of criteria more explicit and precise, that is, to articulate clearly the necessary conceptual commitments entailed by the use of the notion of health. This is what I shall attempt to do, and my primary method will be to determine how we normally use the term in daily conversation, in the ordinary language. If that usage rests, as it clearly does, on an implicit meaning that is significantly different from the medical meaning of health, then this method would seem to be the only appropriate way to draw out that meaning and analyze it.

The objection will be made, of course, that our usage in this society, even if it is distinct from the medical usage, is still a culturally determined meaning and thus can reveal nothing about any inherent, universal understanding of health. I think this objection is not valid for the same reasons that it would not be valid to object that different cultures have significantly different ways of distinguishing between land and water, night and day. The difference between being healthy and unhealthy must be a universal distinction, and although the explanations of that difference will certainly vary widely from culture to culture, too much of social life and human survival depends upon the uniformity of that distinction for it to be significantly culturally dependent. I believe that without doubt my own particular articulation of that difference as it is found in our language will be to some degree culturally biased and subject to criticism, but I also think that the logical structure of the concept of health must necessarily be universal and that our language is as good a place as any to look for it.

CHAPTER TWO

THE PROBLEM OF CRITERIA

Health, as we all know, is one of our overriding considerations. Under normal conditions—that is when we do not need to be constantly concerned with it—we tend to take it for granted, for it is indeed a normal experience and thus not as interesting as war, poverty, injustice, or inflation. But when we do not have it, all these other "more interesting" considerations tend to become less significant, and the less we have of it, the more insignificant they become. Health is not only something we all want; it is a necessary condition for all our other wants to be satisfied. The television commercial may have been oversimplifying when it stated, "If you've got your health, you've got just about everything," but this idea is not obviously ridiculous either. Health, or some degree of it, is at least a fundamental requirement for human life to be worthwhile, and it may even be a characterization of what it means for that life to be worthwhile.

It is interesting, then, that the concept of health has been regarded as so decisively unproblematic as it has by our philosophers and theorists. No body of literature analyzes the meanings and connotations of the term health, its use and misuse, in a fashion comparable to that for other concepts that point to central and desirable things, concepts such as justice, truth, and freedom. If we look at the philosophy journals, we find that the *Philosophers Index*, the standard reference guide, lists only two articles under the heading "Health" from 1968 to 1973, two in 1974, five in 1975, and twelve in 1976. And this only means that the word *health* appeared in the title of the article; in fact, none of these articles is directly concerned with analyzing the concept of health itself. Prior to 1968, the major philosophy index did not even have a subject heading for "Health." Of course, there has always been among certain professional groups, and particularly recently, a thoroughgoing concern with the achievement of health—by doctors with respect to physical functioning, by social scientists with respect to the establishment and adequacy of health care institutions, and by officials with respect to the cost and direction of public health. But, remarkably, the underlying ideas of what health is and what it means to achieve it remain unexplored. Only with respect to the concerns and theories of mental health has the issue even been systematically raised, and here the assumed separation of health into the distinct and essentially autonomous components of mental and physical health has severely limited the conceptual usefulness of the discussion.

The reason for this analytic neglect, of course, is the overwhelming success of the effort to legitimate the biological-medical view of what health is and how to achieve it as the only correct and acceptable conception. The social history of this effort, beginning significantly with the Flexner Report in 1910, has been assembled in many places and is not my concern here (see, for example, Ehrenreich and English; Stevens). This political and institutional effort was greatly aided by the contributions of bio-medical science to the treatment and prevention of diseases. In any case, virtually all discussions of health now assume the medical understanding of the concept, and this understanding is a technical one: health is an objective condition of the body, characterized by proper physiological functioning, a condition that can be scientifically known and therefore technically adjusted and improved in cases of breakdown, just as can the workings of a machine. On this view, health is exclusively a matter of science and biology, a matter of sophisticated physical intervention, whether of surgery or drugs, and therefore can be fully understood and competently practiced only by objectively trained experts, by technicians. Thus, with respect to almost any conceptual or theoretical concern, the idea of health has been decisively confiscated by the doctors and scientists. It is not made the subject of conceptual inquiry because it has been established as an essentially technical term that contains no hidden social or moral implications or ambiguities. The judgment of health, like the judgment of digestible or breathable, is seen as being a desirable, but objectively straightforward and therefore philosophically uninteresting, concern.

This attitude toward the concept of health can be found in the writings of many philosophers and theorists, particularly when they are not concerned with health as an issue but use it as an illustration of a simple, as opposed to a complex, conceptual domain. Thus in the context of a discussion entitled "Is There an Ecological Ethic?" Holmes Rolston III notes in passing:

> It is true, of course, that the means to any end can, in contexts of desperation and urgency, stand in short focus as ultimate values. Air, food, water, health, if we are deprived of them, become at once our concern. Call them ultimate values if you wish, but the ultimacy is instrumental, not intrinsic. We should think him immature whose principal goal was just to breathe, to eat, to drink, to be healthy—merely this and nothing more. (Rolston, p. 98)

In another example, Lisa Newton supports her argument about conservative political theories with this brief and seemingly obvious comment:

> What counts as . . . "health" probably differs from or-
> ganism to organism, and just be *empirically* deter-
> mined for each species by extensive observation. No
> logical difficulties attend such a determination. . . .
> health . . . is an objectively determinable state of my
> body. (Newton, p. 596)

In a discussion of categorical imperatives, philosopher Laslo
Versenyi mentions in passing as another obvious truth that,
with respect to our health, doctors are absolute authorities,
clearly implying that health is only a technical problem:

> A sick man, for example, fearful for his health but to-
> tally unsure of a knowledge of medicine, may rationally
> relinquish his agency with respect to the entire conduct
> of his physical life—diet, exercise, physical activity, etc.
> —to a doctor; and a neurotic may slavishly submit to
> the ruling of his whole physical and mental life by a
> psychiatrist without contradicting his basic purposive-
> ness. And provided that the man is really sick (phys-
> ically and/or mentally) it is perfectly rational and there-
> fore necessary for him as a purposive being to relinquish
> his own concrete agency temporarily or even for the
> rest of his natural life. (Versenyi, p. 269)

All of these examples indicate the completeness and casual-
ness with which philosophers have accepted the medical conception of health. Health is a technical concern, doctors are
the objective experts, and there are no problematic conceptual, moral, or social issues involved. And this perspective is
not even defended or argued, much less considered as a
subject for systematic analysis in itself; it is simply taken for
granted as a clear example to be passingly referred to in
support of arguments about more traditional philosophical
problems.

But can it be this simple? Health is a term that refers to something everybody wants, a universal human good. As Stephen Toulmin puts it while discussing physiology:

> The chief vital functions of the human body are not merely "good in themselves." They are the preconditions for almost any other imaginable human good. . . . Their desirability is evident simply from their status as instruments of good health. (Toulmin, p. 61)

But if health has this significance for human life, should it not also have a more deeply moral, and therefore social, significance? Can it be possible that what is perhaps *the* fundamental human good is only a technical concern with respect to which we can rationally relinquish all control over our lives in deference to a set of objective experts? Terms that characterize basic human goods—terms such as justice, truth, freedom—are generally recognized as moral terms, and philosophers have spent centuries taking moral terms seriously as both conceptually problematic and socially significant. Why is health different? It is an evaluative concept, and as such its use points to the making of a judgment: health is being distinguished from lack of health, or the healthy is being distinguished from the unhealthy. Moreover, it would certainly seem that health is a moral concept in the sense that it can properly be used only to refer to or describe something that is generally and necessarily recognized as valuable. Health is a good thing, something to be desired, and this sense of approval or commendation cannot simply be based on personal whim or idiosyncrasy but is rather linguistic and therefore logical, inherent in the meaning of the term itself. In this sense it would certainly seem similar to moral concepts such as justice, freedom, and good. The normal use of all of these terms commits us to approval

—indeed, it constitutes approval. Perhaps, then, in the absence of a sustained analysis of the moral implications of the concept of health, we should look briefly at what the philosophers have said more generally about moral concepts as such.

Perhaps the central conclusion of modern moral philosophy is the assertion of the categorical distinction between facts and values. Indeed, Philippa Foot suggests: "It would not be an exaggeration to say that the whole of moral philosophy, as it is now widely taught, rests on a contrast between statements of facts and evaluations" (Foot, p. 110). She goes on to characterize the rigorous form of this contrast with respect to the term good, although she herself demurs from it somewhat:

> If a man is given good evidence for a factual conclusion he cannot just refuse to accept the conclusion on the ground that in his scheme of things this evidence is not evidence at all. With evaluations, however, it is different. An evaluation is not connected logically with the factual statements on which it is based. One man may say that a thing is good because of some fact about it, and another may refuse to take that fact as any evidence at all, for nothing is laid down in the meaning of "good" which connects it with one piece of "evidence" rather than another. (pp. 110–111)

R. M. Hare also states this distinction decisively, with no demurral at all:

> If we admit, as I shall later maintain, that it must be part of the function of a moral judgment to prescribe or guide choices, that is to say to entail an answer to some question of the form "What shall I do?"—then it is clear . . . that no moral judgment can be a pure statement of

> fact. . . . The reason why heteronomous principles of
> morality are spurious is that from a series of indicative
> sentences . . . no imperative sentence about what is to
> be done can be derived, and therefore no moral judg-
> ment can be derived from it either. (Hare, 1964, pp.
> 29–30)

Thus, most philosophers agree that moral values cannot be
derived from facts. If we leave aside the murky question
of what constitutes facts, this claim seems straightforward
enough: there can be no concrete empirical evidence from
which one can unequivocally derive a necessary moral judgment.

Now, if a meaningful judgment is to be made using an
evaluative concept such as health or justice, it must be made
on the basis of some set of clear, general, and consistent
criteria. The philosophical problem with evaluative terms
(other than health) has been trying to discover or justify
what that criteria should be. How do we know the good,
the beautiful, the just? What criteria can be convincingly
invoked to legitimate one set of actions directed toward
achieving these goals rather than another? In less complex
societies, the criteria seem to have been rigorously established simply by the strength of tradition. But with the coming of cities and centralized governments, more abstract,
even transcendental, criteria have been needed. For Plato
the necessary criteria could be derived from the Forms; for
Augustine, from the Word of God; for Kant, from Pure Reason; for Adam Smith, from self-interest and the market; and,
more recently, for E. O. Wilson and the sociobiologists,
from evolution. But cynicism has generally prevailed, and
most philosophers now agree that this search for criteria is
really more a linguistic than an empirical or a metaphysical
problem. This is the real force of the fact-value distinction.
Evaluative terms are necessary for human life and language,

and their use entails an absolute commitment to a set of value-laden criteria. That is, the need for definitive value judgments is established linguistically as a necessary dimension of human life, but the particular values, and thus the particular criteria, are established socially and historically and thus are relative and contingent, for there is no Truth about the world that can make them necessary and certain. The values may be felt as absolute, but that is owing to the linguistic imposition of certainty, as well as to the weight of social opinion and the psychological need for conviction. No clear and universal evidence, no empirical facts about the world, can ever entail a specific moral judgment. Thus no decision about what constitutes justice or equality or freedom can ever be derived from what we recognize as scientific knowledge, no matter how detailed or refined. And thus it would seem to follow that the practical meaning of these concepts with respect to the conduct of social life can only be determined culturally and historically, that is, relatively, for we cannot expect to find a final and objective criteria for their use.

Of course, there have been many efforts to do exactly this, to derive a certainty about moral concepts and actions from an objective and unimpeachable given. For most of human history philosophers and moralists have relied upon an appeal to some transcendental source of truth, such as the Forms of Plato or the God of the Christians. Since the rise of science, however, we have accepted the notion that our only hope for certainty about anything lies in achieving objective knowledge about the experienced world, an understanding that leaves the problem of moral concepts in something of a dilemma, since we have also understood that scientific knowledge can never generate moral certainty. Nevertheless, many efforts have been made to derive certain moral principles from objective knowledge about this world, efforts

that have inevitably come down to a claim about the nature
of human nature. For Hobbes it was rational, self-interested,
aggressive, and aquisitive; for Locke, Bentham, and Mill it
was about the same, only somewhat less aggressive; for Kant
it was rational and Protestant; for Marx it was social, productive, and historically rational. These and other theorists
derived various "objective" moral positions from different
versions of human nature, and each such theory has been attacked by others as fundamentally, though not necessarily
intentionally, biased and subjective, since no claim about
human nature has been able to demand universal agreement
and acceptance. One of the most clearly stated of these efforts is John Rawls's A Theory of Justice (1971), and it will be
instructive to look briefly at his assertions and the response
to them as an indication of the traditional mode of discussing
the accepted moral concepts.

As R. M. Hare puts it, Rawls "thinks of a theory of justice
as analogous to a theory in empirical science. It has to square
with what he calls 'facts,' just like, for example, physiological
theories" (Hare, 1975, p. 82). Rawls begins by explicitly putting himself in the tradition of social contract theorists, particularly Locke, Rousseau, and Kant. Like them, Rawls uses
the notion of a social contract as a logical method for isolating
the basic components of objective human nature:

> There is a definite if limited class of facts against which
> conjectured principles can be checked, namely, our
> considered judgments in reflective equilibrium. A the-
> ory of justice is subject to the same rules of method as
> other theories. (Rawls, p. 51)

"Reflective equilibrium" is the imagined condition people
are in when they choose the principles of justice underlying
the social contract. This condition guarantees that they make

their choice absolutely on the basis of their nature as human beings, not on the basis of any historically contingent interests.

> They are the principles that free and rational persons concerned to further their own interests would accept in an initial position of equality as defining the fundamental terms of their association. . . . Among the essential features of this situation is that no one knows his place in society, his class position or social status, nor does any one know his fortune in the distribution of natural assets and abilities, his intelligence, strength, and the like. I shall even assume that the parties do not know their conceptions of the good or their special psychological propensities. The principles of justice are chosen behind a veil of ignorance. This ensures that no one is advantaged or disadvantaged in the choice of principles by the outcome of natural chance or the contingency of social circumstances. (pp. 11–12)

From this effort to abstract the essence of human persons from all specific social situations, Rawls arrives at the "general facts" that can generate, through hypothetical choices, objective principles of justice. Just what these principles are exactly is not our concern here, although, as it turns out, they are essentially a restatement of the values of a liberal and individualistic society. But Rawls's method of deriving moral certainty from a universal claim about the objective facts of human nature is fully representative of most modern attempts to establish definitively the correct criteria for the use of moral concepts, and thus the criteria for social and political judgments.

> The principles of their actions do not depend upon social or natural contingencies, nor do they reflect the

bias of the particulars of their plan of life or the aspirations that motivate them. By acting from these principles persons express their nature as free and equal rational beings subject to the general conditions of human life. (pp. 252–253)

Also, these principles are objective (Rawls, p. 516).

The response to these assertions from Rawls's philosophical colleagues has been equally representative of the discussion of moral concepts. Almost uniformly, they point out that his derivation is not objective but rests fundamentally on hidden assumptions and subjective bias. Thomas Nagel comments:

It is a fundamental feature of Rawls' conception of the fairness of the original position that it should not permit the choice of principles of justice to depend on a particular conception of the good over which the parties may differ. The construction does not, I think, accomplish this, and there are reasons to believe it cannot be successfully carried out. . . . The original position seems to presuppose not just a neutral theory of the good, but a liberal, individualistic conception. (Nagel, pp. 8–10)

Milton Fisk shares this view:

Thus on the basis of the atomistic human nature of Rawls' original position we derive, not surprisingly, atomistic conclusions that are not sufficient for community and seem incompatible with it. . . . The supporting conception of human nature loses its claim to social and historical neutrality. (Fisk, p. 67)

Concerning Rawls's basic argument in support of objectivity, R. M. Hare finds that he "is here advocating a kind of sub-

jectivism, in the narrowest and most old-fashioned sense"
(Hare, 1975, p. 82), and H. L. A. Hart feels that at least one
of Rawls's main arguments fails because "he does harbor a
latent ideal of his own," an ideal that "powerfully impreg-
nates [his] book at many points" and that "is, of course,
among the chief ideals of Liberalism" (Hart, p. 252). Gerald
Dworkin sums up the logic of these responses by adding his
own criticisms "to those arguments . . . that show how many
of the substantive claims that emerge from hypothetical con-
tractualism follow only because implicit and controversial assumptions are built in a non-obvious fashion into the structure of the theory" (Dworkin, p. 139).

The case against the objectivity of Rawls's principles is convincing, and it is not hard to see that any such claim con-
necting the facts of human nature to the definitive meaning
of moral concepts must include a reliance on surreptitious
values. Rawls attempts to elucidate the objective criteria for
understanding and instituting justice, and his analysis depends explicitly upon a putative straightforward and noncontroversial conception of what human beings are and will do
as such, abstracted away from all particular historical con-
tingencies. But he describes this conception repeatedly as
being one of free, equal, and rational beings: when people
are in a pure state of freedom, equality, and rationality, he
claims, it is factually clear that they will choose objective
principles of justice. Thus we need only imagine those conditions, analyze the consequences, and justice can be objectively defined. In other words, the argument about the
objective criteria for justice depends fundamentally upon a
prior and unargued claim about the seemingly standard and
universal criteria for freedom, equality, and rationality. But
why should we assume that the concepts of freedom and
equality, for example, are any less problematic than justice?
Why not rather derive the meaning of freedom from an as-

sumption about the meanings of justice and truth? Rawls's lengthy and complex argument asserting the objectivity of one moral concept depends finally upon a hidden and unsupported assumption about the objectivity of other moral concepts. His "facts" turn out in the end to be value judgments.

Rawls is not alone in this mistake, for any attempt to derive necessary moral principles from the facts of human nature must impose an uninspected moral content on those facts. Since Hobbes, all moral and political theories have assumed that one or more moral concepts, such as natural freedom or natural rationality, can be used to describe simply and unambiguously a universal given of human life, an objective certainty from which moral consequences flow. And it is this type of argument that the fact-value distinction is meant to critique. The fact-value distinction rests absolutely on the idea that an empirical or scientific fact contains no hidden moral message whatsoever; thus, no moral instructions, no criteria for the use of moral concepts, can be derived from it. By their very nature, moral concepts entail direction and commitment; they necessitate action and involvement. If the principles of their application could be definitively derived from undeniable evidence, our political and economic life, as well as our daily and personal interactions, would be decisively affected, for some sort of moral unity where there is now moral diversity would be entailed. The fact-value distinction requires that such a derivation is impossible and suggests that moral values must ultimately be based on such things as cultural bias, personal history, and the interests of power, since no objectively binding standard can ever be found.

Later, we shall look more carefully at the effort to derive moral criteria from the notion of a universal human nature. But from this brief look at Rawls's attempt to understand justice we can see that, according to the main philosophical tradition, moral concepts can only be defined, or even legitimately discussed, in terms of other moral concepts, never in terms of empirical and objective facts. Thus, to the degree that the concept of health refers to an objective and factual state of the body, it cannot, it seems, represent a moral concept in any traditional sense. On the other hand, to the degree that it is considered to be in any sense a moral term, as it often is in discussions of mental health, it must be understood as unconnected to objective, empirical facts. This conceptual requirement accounts for, as we shall see, much of the elaborate theoretical gulf between our medical ideas of physical health and our psychoanalytic ideas of mental health. But, as everyone agrees, the judgment of mental health is a complex, confused, and culturally biased effort— in which the concept of health, indeed, may not even apply (cf. Szasz, 1970). The judgment of physical health, however, according to the medical view, is both the paradigmatic use of the concept of health and a judgment that can finally rest on technical and empirical information.

CHAPTER THREE

THE MEDICAL VIEW

The Body as Morally Neutral

Now, if moral concepts can only be discussed in terms of other moral concepts, then the philosophers' neglect of the concept of health begins to seem more understandable. For does not the judgment of health, or being healthy, differ somewhat from this description of moral concepts? Is it not clear, at least on the face of it, that the evaluation of health is indeed logically connected with the factual statements on which it is based? When a doctor, for example, describes someone as healthy, it would seem that he or she is directly referring to empirical, even scientific, facts. Indeed, this must be the case even when those of us who are not doctors describe our friends or relatives as healthy. Although we may be mistaken—that is, they may have an illness we do not know about—so may doctors, and our lay judgments, like their professional ones, are based on direct empirical evidence of healthlike activity, activity that would more or less generally and universally be recognized as justifying at least the judgment of good physical health. Philosophers do not regard this empirical reference of the judgment of health as contradicting the fact-value distinction; in fact, they recognize and embrace it willingly. Stephen Toulmin, for example, directly identifies the "vital functions of the human body," which he attests throughout his essay are empirically and scientifically knowable, as the "instruments of good health," perhaps the most fundamental of all human goods (Toulmin,

p. 61). Here a straightforward moral evaluation—a human
good—is being derived directly from the functions of the
body as they are understood by medical science. As Toulmin
puts it, "their desirability is evident simply from their status
as the instruments of good health." He makes this connection even clearer in other passages:

> The logical gulf between "facts" and "values" has little
> practical significance for either medicine or medical sci-
> ence. . . . Either way, the *rational* significance of vital
> organization or functioning is inseparable from its *eth-
> ical* significance. (p. 62)

> The nature of *health* is, at one and the same time, a
> matter for empirical discovery and a matter of evalua-
> tive decision. (p. 65)

Yet Toulmin is not arguing that values can be derived
from facts:

> If the basic empirical subject-matter of [modern physi-
> ology] were composed merely of biophysical and bio-
> chemical processes, directly explicable in terms of gen-
> eral laws and physical necessities, we might perhaps
> declare physiology indifferent as between the evalua-
> tive conceptions of "health" and "disease." (p. 61)

Rather, he makes the claim, a common one among those
who address the issue at all, that health is a *special kind* of
value, one with none of the social and political implications
of recognized moral terms.

> Instead, modern physiology is intelligible only in terms
> of the same "organic systems" that lie at the base of
> medicine: systems whose existence and character are
> defined in terms of the functions they serve. As a re-

sult, the logical gulf between "facts" and "values" has
little practical significance for either medicine or medical science. (p. 62)

That is, the facts about physiology give the value of health a
clear empirical base, so that we can neither argue with the
facts nor deny the value. The argument goes something like
this. With respect to the body, health is a good thing in the
same way that, with respect to a piano, being in tune is a
good thing. Both are machines whose purposes can be fulfilled only if they are functioning properly; therefore, in
terms of the machine, functioning properly is a good thing.
However, all other human purposes and values depend so
intimately upon the proper functioning of the body, in ways
they do not depend upon the proper functioning of a piano
or any other machine, that the health of the body is an
absolute good thing, whereas the proper functioning of all
other machines can only be judged as good relative to more
fundamental human values.

   This argument appears reasonable and seems to accord
with common sense. It can even be defended linguistically,
since we use the concept health directly to evaluate the
working of the body but only indirectly and metaphorically,
with irony and humor, to evaluate the working of man-made
machines. The connection, then, is between the centrality of
the human body, the biological facts of its processes, and the
consequent necessity of the desirability of health for all human beings.

   For us today, the mere number of individual atoms and
   cells in the body is a secondary matter. Its complexity is
   chiefly systemic and functional; and, to the extent that
   its value and intelligibility alike spring from that same
   systemic character, we have no choice whether to pre-
   fer normal to pathological working, function to dysfunction, health to disease. (Toulmin, p. 62)

Thus, the special status of the body in human life confers a
special status on the concept of health in human action and
consciousness. Like the concepts of justice, freedom, truth,
and good, it is an evaluative term that demands support linguistically, but unlike them, it has a clear and unambiguous
empirical referent. We can all agree, as we cannot with the
other concepts, on what health is, on how to recognize it,
and on the fact that we must all strive to achieve it, for
ourselves necessarily and for others morally. (Interestingly,
whereas it seems relatively easy for a society to justify organized efforts to kill people for the sake of social goals, it appears far more difficult to justify organized efforts to make
people unhealthy for the sake of social goals.) From this
perspective it is clear that as a moral term, health has a
very special status. I have quoted Toulmin's arguments as
both clear and representative of the common understanding
of health as it is used and discussed today by the professionals
who address it, whether doctors or medical theorists. Bodily
health is recognized as a universal good and as the legitimate
subject of intense scientific and empirical study. Since the
rise of scientific medicine, doctors have not only been convinced of their certain knowledge of what health is, or at
least when it is missing, but have also been taught and have
accepted the idea that the healing of the body takes precedence over all other social and political values.

It is not so much the fact of the special status of health but
the conceptual and moral consequences of this status that are
interesting. Health is recognized as a value that has a logical,
intrinsic relationship to empirical facts, but in spite of or,
more likely, because of this, it is also treated as a value that
has no logical, intrinsic relationship to social and political
morality. That is, nothing about how people should act in society, how they should organize politically, how they should
treat one another (other than curing the ill) can be derived
from an acceptance of the universal value of health. Health

may be a universal good, but the application of this good is
limited to the functioning of the body; no other moral knowledge can be derived from it. In this way, of course, it is
even more decisively separated from other moral terms, such
as justice, equality, and freedom, terms that have obvious
social and political implications and have been at the center
of much moral debate and confusion. Such terms, it has
been decided, have no straightforward empirical referent, so
there is no final and accurate way to choose between one
idea of justice and another, between one idea of freedom and
another. Any such choice must finally come down to matters
of definition and perspective, and there are good arguments
on each side. Health, on the other hand, has a clear empirical referent, but, the argument goes, our certain knowledge
of the determinants, the criteria, for health can never help
us in our search for justice, freedom, or the good life. If
health is a moral concept, it is an unusual one and consequently is of little help to us with our fundamental moral
concerns.

Statements of this position are not hard to find, and once
again Toulmin is perhaps the clearest. First he identifies
physiology, as opposed to biology, as the value-laden medical study of bodily health. Then he argues that, with respect
to health, the empirical facts of physiology virtually determine our actions:

> In medicine, as in law, we face choices and decisions
> that can be made conscientiously, only in the light
> of the best empirical understanding we can command;
> and, once it is sufficiently complete, this empirical
> understanding commonly leaves us precious little room
> for real choice. (Toulmin, p. 65)

But with respect to broader social and political choices, even
those having to do with the delivery of health care, physiology and the value of health are no help:

> So, let me ask: if we start with the living totality of
> medicine, and make a move to the abstraction called
> "physiology," what do we leave out in the course of that
> abstraction? The answer is: all concern with values and
> choices *other than* those intrinsic to the concepts of
> medical science itself—all concern with questions about
> the social context of medicine; about priorities in the
> availability of health care; about whose welfare our ac-
> cumulated medical understanding is to be applied to
> promote, for what price; about the political role of the
> medical profession, and so on. . . . (pp. 65–66)

René Dubos goes even further, finding an inevitable conflict between ethics and medicine as the empirical study of
health.

> Only biomedical science can provide the knowledge re-
> quired for policies of collective medical control neces-
> sary for survival in the modern world. (Dubos, p. 127)

> Everyone agrees that scientific knowledge and technical
> competence are not sufficient for the practice of medi-
> cine. . . . Medical ethics is concerned primarily with
> the trust placed by the patient in his doctor and in-
> volves moral judgments. The professional and ethical
> responsibilities of the physician are not limited to the
> patient entrusted to his care; they extend to the society
> in which he lives and to mankind in general. (p. 134)

> Conflicts between medical progress and medical ethics
> appear in almost all aspects of the science and practice
> of medicine. . . . Thus, a strict and legalistic interpreta-
> tion of medical ethics almost inevitably stands in the
> way of medical progress. This state of affairs is not pe-
> culiar of medicine; it applies just as well to other types
> of technological innovations. . . . (p. 137)

Thus, although the science of medicine can best contribute
to good health, it cannot generate moral social actions and,

indeed, will inevitably conflict with those actions. Medicine is empirical and therefore technological; its use must be determined by technical, not moral, judgment.

This notion of medicine takes for granted that health is both a general good, and an empirical and technical concern, one that is unconnected to the moral issues of social and political life. It is important to remember that these theorists are assuming, not supporting or defending, their belief that the concept of health works in this way. The depth of this assumption and the casual manner with which it is asserted, when it is even recognized, can be shown through an analysis of a statement by H. Tristram Engelhardt, Jr., who is both a doctor and a philosopher.

> Health is a normative term but not in the sense of a moral virtue. Though health is a good, and though it may be morally praiseworthy to try to be healthy and to advance the health of others, still, all things being equal, it is a misfortune, not a misdeed, to lack health. Health is more an aesthetic than an ethical term; it is more beauty than virtue. Thus, one does not condemn someone for no longer being healthy, though one may sympathize with him over the loss of a good. (Engelhardt, p. 126)

In this passage, the opening discussion in an essay titled "The Concepts of Health and Disease," Engelhardt attempts to deny health its moral status while recognizing its normative, that is, its evaluative, use. This, of course, is the crucial issue. Health is a good, but if it can be established as being exclusively an instrumental, technical good, then it will not carry significant moral weight, and its empirical referent will not be a moral problem. All other positions, indeed all modern discussions of health, rest on this argument, for it is the only way in which health can be understood as both a judgment of value and as the subject of scientific knowledge if the fact-value distinction is to remain inviolate. If health were to be accepted as having a moral significance greater than that of, say, beauty (which it would certainly seem to have on the face of it), a moral significance similar to that of freedom or justice, then either health could no longer be the subject of an empirical medical *science* or some of our most crucial and cherished philosophical and *moral*, not to say political, assumptions would have to be drastically over-hauled. Depending upon the extent of the moral significance, the entire discussion of health care, perhaps even of politics and economics, would be affected. At the very least, the idea of the doctor's responsibility to the patient and to society could no longer be defined strictly in terms of the biology and physiology of the body, as is suggested by the medical model.

Clearly, Engelhardt's argument is important; the problem is that it is simply wrong. That is, his position may be valid (though I do not think so and will attempt to disprove it), but his argument cannot be correct, for it does not distinguish between a moral or ethical term and an aesthetic or technical one. This is evident if we simply substitute "freedom" for "health" in his discussion. Freedom, I believe, is without question a moral and ethical term, and yet Engelhardt's argument equally distinguishes it from virtue. Freedom is a good, it is praiseworthy to try to be free, and it is a misfortune, not a misdeed, to lack freedom. This is equally true, for example, of having justice (as opposed to being just). Thus, unless it is also true that freedom and justice are not ethical terms, his argument is necessarily specious. Yet this very speciousness, and the cavalier assurance with which the error is committed, indicates both the strength and seeming naturalness of the accepted conception, as well as the crucial importance attached to the need for such a conception to be convincing.

Health, then, has been treated as something that is a good

thing, that is empirically grounded, and that does not raise
basic moral issues about social life. Within these assumptions
and limitations, doctors and philosophers have discussed and
analyzed health as though it were a concern of natural science that could be defined fully through its location in biological or physical theory. Its meaning may be in some ways
theoretically obscure, but that is regarded as a matter for
scientists to discuss, not philosophers, since as a technical
term its analysis offers no significant insights into human life
or consciousness.

This conception is a reflection of the mind-body dualism
that continues to permeate Western science and philosophy
(see below, Conclusion). It lies at the base of modern medicine and has informed the singleminded medical effort to
achieve health by repairing and correcting, through surgical
and chemical intervention, the body's mechanisms. The necessary translation from this conception of health to the practice of medical science has been made through the abstracted
idea that the body has its own empirical laws and processes
that work independently of mental or social life. The body,
then—as opposed to the human being—becomes the locus of
health, and the conception that health has no moral impact
is secure. Since the body and its mechanisms are completely
self-contained, they are available for the physician to treat—
that is, to repair—as best as possible whenever they break
down. Toulmin, once again, makes this clear through his
conception of the vital functions of life, of which physiology
is the science:

> [The physician's] whole enterprise is nowadays intel-
> ligible, and capable of being rationally expounded, only
> in terms of a systemic picture of vital organization and
> functioning; and this picture presupposes the existence
> and integrity of all the main functioning systems in the
> human frame. (Toulmin, p. 61)

Since it should be clear to all of us, including Dr. Toulmin, that the human frame must also intake food, breathe air, and get exercise, not to mention have some kind of satisfactory social interaction, in order to maintain those vital functions, it should seem rather arbitrary that this idea of functioning is conceptualized as limited to and contained in the body. Should the "systemic picture of vital organization and functioning" that makes the physician's enterprise "intelligible and capable of being rationally expounded" not also at least presuppose "the existence and integrity of all the main functioning systems" of the larger ecological context with which the body must necessarily interact? Perhaps it should even include the social context. These seem to be obvious points, particularly the former, and yet once again the ease with which they are ignored, the certainty with which the interior of the body is assumed to be the decisive locus of medical science, and thus of health, indicates the extent of the uncritical commitment to the medical approach to health. Once again Dr. Engel captures the nature of this uncritical commitment and its consequences for human health:

> In spite of its underlying reductionism and dualism, it is nonetheless undeniable that, as a scientific framework within which to elaborate the disordered bodily mechanisms involved in disease, the biomedical model has been extraordinarily fruitful. Unfortunately, this success has served not only to entrench dualism and reductionism but also to encourage more enthusiastic advocates of the biomedical model to promote it as ultimately capable of explaining all aspects of health and disease. The dogmatism inherent in such blind faith in, and exaggerated claims for, the model has been a powerful factor in deflecting scientific interest and attention from problems that do not readily yield to the biomedical approach. Outstandingly neglected areas are the

more personal, human, psychological and social aspects
of health and disease, and the caring rather than the
curing functions of the physician. These biomedicine
considers neither accessible to rigorous scientific evaluation nor essential for the education of the physician.
(Engel, p. 258)

The body-centered, body-limited medical model has been
and remains today the defining paradigm for our professional and philosophical conceptions of health and for medical training, medical practice, and the funding of medical
research. For all of its conceptual abstraction, it has the
effect, since a particular body is always connected with a
particular, living person, of making virtually all our efforts in
health care strongly centered on the individual. When someone is unhealthy, it can only mean that his or her body has
broken down, and the only rational procedure is to attempt
to treat or "cure" that person as an isolated, independent
individual. The only legitimate response to bad health, we
are told, is for the doctor as a technician to treat the individual as a body. In this way it is possible for the practice of
medicine, like the conception of health, to be understood as
both moral and nonmoral. It is moral in the sense that keep-
ing the body functioning is a universal moral good, but somehow it is still only a technical good, and thus the doctor's actions as a doctor have no larger social or political meaning.
In his well-received book, *The Logic of Medicine*, Dr.
Edmond O. Murphy of the Johns Hopkins Medical School,
undertakes in over 300 densely written pages

to explore the ideas behind the evaluation of the sources
and interpretations of the data from which the corpus of
medical knowledge is to be derived. The facts, I hope,
are true: but this is not what matters. Biological mechanisms are complex and what purports to be a fact has a

"short half-life." The rules of evidence are more durable
and it seems all the more strange that so little attention
is paid to them. (Murphy, p. 3)

Dr. Murphy proceeds to discuss, through complex and refined arguments, such matters as classification, inference,
syllepsis, indeterminacy, and causality, but he gives absolutely no consideration to such concerns as social relationships, social institutions, culture, morality, or politics. Indeed, no such terms even appear in the index.

Another effect of this body-individual idea of health is that
whenever someone begins to discuss the concept of health,
he or she almost inevitably winds up discussing the concept
of disease. Disease refers to a breakdown of the body, and
throughout the literature on health it is treated as the opposite of health. Thus the discussion of health quickly becomes
the discussion of disease, a conceptual maneuver that successfully skirts any real analysis of health as a moral judgment. For example, Engelhardt spends the first page of his
essay discussing the concept of health and the next thirteen
pages discussing the concept of disease. The same is true of
Dubos in his chapter "The Determinants of Health and Disease," only in his case the numbers are two pages as opposed
to twenty-three. And the examples can be multiplied. As
Dr. Chester R. Burns comments, "the view of health as the
logical opposite of disease [is a] fundamental legac[y] in the
philosophies of Western medical science" (Burns, 1975, p.
20).

Recently, however, some new and more integrative conceptions of health and health care have been put forward.
The systemic involvement of the human body with the human person associated with that body, with the larger ecological system, and even in some cases with a social system is
recognized, and the exclusive identification of health with

the physiology of the body is rejected. Even such an austere-sounding concern as the World Health Organization has, in the preamble to its charter, announced that "Health is a state of complete physical, mental, and social well-being and not merely the absence of disease or infirmity." These new conceptions, ranging from holistic and humanistic concerns with new techniques of health maintenance, such as bio-feedback, acupuncture, meditation, nutrition, and vitamins, to more radical critiques of the relation between medicine and health are quite interesting, and three points need to be made about them. First, they are obviously a response to a felt lacuna in the medical conception and to a perceived failure in medical practice. Increasing numbers of people are recognizing that health, as they understand it and expect it, is not being addressed or achieved by the medical profession. Second, these integrative approaches to health have been generally received by the medical profession with hostility, scorn, and dismissal. Though some doctors have shown interest and a few have fully accepted and developed certain of the new techniques, the medical establishment—meaning the majority of doctors, the American Medical Association, the government funding agencies, and, particularly, the medical schools—have remained uninterested and even contemptuous. In other words, these approaches are not seen as valuable ideas and positive directions for improved health care in the way that, say, a cure for cancer or a new technique for birth control would be. Rather, they are generally perceived as practical and theoretical threats to the established medical conception of human health.

Third, despite the insular attitude of the medical powers, most holistic, and even radical, approaches share a basic conceptual assumption with the medical model. That is, they center the locus of health on the individual: the individual must take more responsibility for his or her actions with respect to health, in the sense of knowing what to eat, getting the right exercise, introspection, and the like. Whereas the doctors have made health into a matter of adjusting the mechanisms of the individual body, a matter in which the conscious individual is generally not involved, the humanists have stressed the idea that health is a matter of conscious individual choices. Thus, both the humanists and the doctors tend to deny conceptually that health is a social, and thus a moral, issue. The domain of health has been expanded to include the physical context and environment of physiological functions, but the question of health as a moral judgment relating to social and political life, for all the implicit and explicit critiques of medical practice and the medical model, is still not being raised.

Dubos, whose book, according to its back cover, addresses "The Whole Man and his Total Environment," makes his holistic approach clear:

> Clinical and epidemiological studies show that the inextricably interrelated body, mind, and environment must be considered together in any medical situation whether it involves a single patient or a whole community. (Dubos, p. 85)

But his later definition of health shows more exactly how he means this approach to be interpreted:

> Health will be considered in the following pages . . . not as an ideal state of well-being achieved through the complete elimination of disease, but as a modus vivendi enabling imperfect men to achieve a rewarding and not too painful existence while they cope with an imperfect world. In this light, health cannot be defined in the absolute, because different persons expect such different things from life. A Wall Street executive, a lumber-

> jack in the Canadian Rockies, a newspaper boy at a
> crowded street corner, a steeplechase jockey, a clois-
> tered monk, and the pilot of a supersonic combat plane
> have various physical and mental needs. The imperfec-
> tions and limitations of the flesh and of the mind do not
> have equal importance for them. (p. 88)

With respect to an understanding of health, Dubos is taking
the social order absolutely for granted. He treats the job
structure, the class structure, the differential opportunity,
even the implied sexism as independent givens that the health
professions must take into account just as they would the
bone structure or the circulation of the blood. It does not
seem quite as clear as he assumes that different people expect different things from life or that they have different
physical and mental needs, but it is absolutely clear that
people from different class or educational or occupational
backgrounds in our society will have very different possibilities of satisfying their physical and mental needs. For
Dubos, it seems, the "inextricably interrelated body, mind,
and environment" simply does not include social life. Among
the holistic critics of modern medicine, Dubos is perhaps the
most committed to biomedical science as the final arbiter of
health, and thus his approach to the subject is essentially
technical and professional, though on a grander social and
environmental scale:

> Physicians must learn to work with engineers, ar-
> chitects, and general biologists, as well as with city
> planners, lawyers, and politicians responsible for the
> management of our social life. Only through such col-
> laboration can they help society ward off, insofar as
> possible, dangers to physical and mental health inher-
> ent in all technological and social changes. . . . (Dubos,
> p. 117)

The technical orientation is clear: doctors need only expand their technical manipulations in conjunction with other technicians and controllers.

Far more radical in their interpretation of this environmental position and more critical of medical science are the analysts Ivan Illich and Rick Carlson. Yet here again, health is discussed as primarily a technical problem. Illich and Carlson believe that the ordinary individual must take primary and personal responsibility for his or her health through essentially autonomous actions and knowledge, for the doctors and scientists are more of a threat than a help. According to Illich, in his widely recognized book, *Medical Nemesis*:

> "Health," after all, is simply an everyday word that is used to designate the intensity with which individuals cope with their internal states and their environmental conditions. (Illich, p. 7)

> Health is a task, and as such is not comparable to the physiological balance of beasts. Success in this personal task is in large part the result of the self-awareness, self-discipline, and inner resources by which each person regulates his own daily rhythm and actions, his diet, and his sexual activity. (pp. 273–274)

And in *The End of Medicine*, Carlson stresses the individual by distinguishing between two kinds of knowledge:

> There is the need for information—what to do about one signal or another, when to ask for help, what kinds of food to eat . . . and so on. But of equal importance is experiential knowledge—body consciousness—the capacity to read the topography of feelings and sensations. . . . The second takes nothing less than the assumption by the individual of the responsibility for health, and

> concomitantly an escape from a dependency on others.
> A healer can only help to restore health and maintain it.
> The individual is chiefly responsible. . . . The pursuit of
> health is not limited to heroes. Although we know little
> about health, what we do know is easy to execute and is
> largely dependent upon the individual. (Carlson, p. 187)

All these theorists criticize the narrowness of modern medicine, and all of them mention the "socioenvironmental" context and note that something should probably be done about it. But, like the doctors and philosophers they criticize, they view the concept of health as being relevant only to the body, the individual, and physiological processes. The context has been expanded beyond the human frame just enough to make it reasonable to suggest that either the doctors need technical help or they are just on the wrong track and the individual must take over. Though the categorical emphasis on the body has been mitigated to some degree, the stress on the individual and on techniques remains. The issue of health as a moral concept available for and applicable to the judgment of social and political life is still not addressed. And yet the positions taken assume that this apparent moral dimension either has been or can be rejected, for otherwise health cannot be an exclusively technical and personal concern. It appears that so long as health is understood as essentially a property of individuals and their physical life, it will continue to fall on the body side of the mind-body dualism, and our practical and conceptual approaches to it will remain technical and individualistic.

But is there another possibility? Surely, even obviously, health *is* a property of bodies, individuals, and physiological processes. The issue is not *whether* this is the case, but whether this is *all* that is the case. I have been arguing that the traditional assumption, even the assumption of many of

the recent critics of medicine, is that this *is* all there is, that
health can be fully understood and discussed in these terms.
One group of critics, however, manifestly rejects this assumption. The Marxists—social scientists, together with a
few doctors—use a Marxist analysis of capitalist economy to
argue that the issues of health and illness are systematically
connected with the market institutions of production, class,
and control. Most typically, they attempt to demonstrate
how structural requirements for power and profit dramatically skew the distribution of health care services away from
the poor and needy toward the rich and powerful. This approach, taken explicitly by the Health-PAC group (a group of
doctors and researchers who publish critical reports on the
health industry) and Vincente Navarro and more implicitly
by Robert Alford, is much more an analysis of institutions
than of health as such and consequently apparently takes
for granted, always implicitly and seemingly by default, the
medical view of what constitutes health.

Another group of Marxists, however, is beginning to apply
social and economic theory to the development of a more
systematic critique of medical practice with respect to the
incidence of illness and the breakdown of health in capitalist
society. This group, represented by Lesley Doyal in England and by Joe Eyer, Evan Stark, and Peter Schnall and
Rochelle Kern in America, is concerned with how the normal workings of a capitalist economy systemically make
people ill, particularly the workers, the women, the aged,
and the minorities. The Americans taking this approach are
semiorganized and have articulated a theoretical position
they call historical materialist epidemiology (HME). According to John Bradley,

> the fundamental proposition of materialist epidemiol-
> ogy is that any realistic discussion of health must focus

attention first on the social relations of production and
reproduction in the society. Alongside medicine and
public health, materialist epidemiology puts the workplace, community and home at the root of the struggle
for health and clarifies the role these play in causing,
perpetrating, and/or preventing ill health. (Bradley, p.
17)

As a theoretical position, HME points toward an understanding of the relationships between institutions, environment, and health, relationships that are, I believe, critical to
any adequate conceptualization of health. In Chapter 6 I shall
discuss these relationships at some length, and there, as well
as throughout, I am indebted to the research, insights, and
analytic perspectives of these Marxist theorists. (Indeed, in
many ways I consider this book itself to be in large part a
philosophical clarification of the social and analytic issues
they raise.) However, despite their apparently thoroughgoing
rejection of the individual-centered medical model, these
analysts still share, if only because of their avoidance or
unawareness of the issue, a fundamental conceptual orientation with the more traditional theorists of health and medicine. That is, they still speak of health as though it were a
clearly defined, nonproblematic term, one that needs no systematic analysis and one that they can refer to at will, along
with all other commentators, even the proponents of, in
their view, the most fraudulent theories. Implicitly, at least,
the Marxists, like all other users of the term, must define
their own version of health, and in their case it seems to be
something like the condition in which most of us would more
or less be if we were not subject to the oppressive institutions of capitalist society. Thus Schnall and Kern remark,
"This struggle between workers and owners . . . has . . .
significant consequences on the health of workers and their
families" (Schnall and Kern, p. 105), and Doyal comments,

"Ill health cannot, therefore, be attributed simply to capitalism in any crude sense. On the other hand, we cannot make sense of the patterns of health and illness outside the context of the mode of production in which they occur" (Doyal, p. 27).

Statements like these illustrate an effort to conceptualize health in a larger social context than either the physical body or individual actions. Nevertheless, without a deeper analysis of the concept itself, the term can only be implicitly understood in one of two senses: either it is a concept defined by the theory itself, in which case it becomes simply a Marxist category and the entire Marxist argument with respect to health reduces to a tautology or becomes noncommunicable, since no one else defines health that way; or the term must be defined independently of Marxist theory so that the logical and empirical relationships between a Marxist analysis and the concept of health can be demonstrated, in which case it becomes necessary to state this independent definition clearly. But since this independent definition is not clearly stated, and since we can also assume that the Marxists do not intend their argument to be either tautologous or noncommunicable, we can only conclude that their use of the term health refers to what they understand to be a clear and established meaning—and of course the only such meaning immediately available for theoretical and academic use is that of the medical model. In other words, by both using the term so forcefully and not offering an alternative conceptualization (the need for which, by the way, is far more consciously recognized and attempted by the holistic health advocates), these epidemiological Marxists must by default accept that their historical materialist critique of the medical model logically reduces to the claim that poverty, working conditions, sexism, and environmental pollution make people physically ill.

Undeniably, these are important claims, and, as Schnall and Kern indicate, much epidemiological research into these connections needs to be done. On the other hand, such claims are not unique, they do not require an elaborate Marxist theoretical structure to make them apparent, and they are not generally opposed, though they are largely ignored by capitalist institutions, which, of course, is one of the central points of these investigators. As a result, although these theorists are indeed making important contributions to the discussions of health in modern society, contributions that I feel are unique and necessary both for their scope and their commitment, they are not as yet successfully making what is clearly their major and most critical argument: namely, that our generally unquestioned acceptance, as a society, of the scientific-medical approach to health results in severe social and institutional magnitudes of illness and suffering. Unlike other commentators on the issue of health, these Marxist analysts have a social and political perspective deeply embedded in their theoretical apparatus, but like other commentators, they finally rely on an implicit notion of health that can only be made explicit by reference to the biophysiological conceptualization of medicine. Because of this, they cannot make a fundamental critique of medical practice but can only point out overlooked connections among independent events. Unfortunately, it is probably in large part their historical materialist approach that leaves them in this dilemma, for although it is obviously a critical and necessary method for social analysis, it is not one that has traditionally raised as· a central issue the analysis and evaluation of concepts. And in this case, because of the depth to which the medical concepts are embedded in our understanding, it is this analysis and evaluation that must take precedence over evidence of historical patterns or empirical relationships in any critical discussion of health in our society.

The Marxists wish to use the concept of health as a moral and political term, but they do little to establish it as such other than to express their apparent sense of anger and injustice. Thus despite their thoroughgoing social perspective, the essential dilemma remains: health, according to the medical understanding, is a technical term referring to physical functioning, but it also seems to carry moral weight, and it is often used, as we have seen, in just this way. The conflict is obviously there, but it is seldom noted analytically, since by far the preponderance of modern authority and agreement is on the side of the technical-medical view.

On the other hand, findings in the developing field of medical anthropology give support to my arguments on the other side, for much of the work being done in this area is necessarily oriented to demonstrating the intrinsic moral and social aspects of tribal notions and practices with regard to health. In one of the major studies from this emerging discipline, Horacio Fabrega and Daniel Silver comment on the attitudes toward health and illness within the Mayan community of Zinacantan, a township of Mexican Indians in the State of Chiapas, Mexico.

> In Zinacanteco thought, illness is seen as reflecting and expressing the status of a man's relations with himself, his social group, and his deities. For example, hostility and envy, two feelings that can pervade and structure interpersonal relations, are believed to be the motivations that lead others to promote illness and injury. . . . Similarly, transgressions of the spiritual and/or social code are believed to be punished by divinely sent illness. The individual himself, his worldly contemporaries, and the gods are locked in a triple web of relationships; and a frequent expression of disarticulation in this web is illness, or *chamel*. It is in this sense that one can speak of illness in Zinacantan as having a moral

basis: the individual's essentially sacred and spiritual
view of himself and others requires that he behave ap-
propriately and in conformance with socially validated
rules; but chamel both reflects and symbolizes a disar-
ticulation of this triple balance. (Fabrega and Silver, p.
81)

In a study of the Fipa in southwest Tanzania, R. G. Willis
describes the role and responsibilities of the tribal doctor:

The task of a Fipa doctor in a case of "serious" illness is
to identify and drive out the intrusive agency which is
causing the sickness, and so enable his client to re-
establish at once both the internal economy of his body
and his external economy as a social being. . . . Persons
seeking to improve their situation within the larger,
interpersonal system of exchange tend to go to a doctor.
(Willis, p. 148)

These studies and others show that in many other cultures
health and illness are traditionally deeply intertwined, conceptually and practically, with the social, moral, and political
life of the community. Indeed, it seems apparent that this,
rather than our, view has been historically the normal way of
thinking about health. It has even been suggested by Robin
Horton and Peter Morley, among others, that our culture, or
at least the patients in our culture, also thinks about health in
this way, only we do not realize it, being so thoroughly
mystified by the scientific credibility of the medical model.

Rarely has the esoterica of Western medicine and science percolated down to the commonsense level of
reality without a concomitant dilution of factual content
and the incorporation of some degree of mysticism and
"magic." Thus, while modern industrial man submits to
the scientifically-based *materia medica* of the allopathic

physician, it does not necessarily follow that the former understands either the knowledge behind medical practice and its nosology, or the complexity of treatments offered him by the latter. In essence, the allopath's patient is, like the Zande, a participant in a belief system. Perhaps the essential difference is that the Azande are more involved in, and less mystified by, both the belief system itself and the diagnostic utterances of its practitioners than are the patients within the Western allopathic medical context. (Morley, p. 15)

Insights such as these have led some anthropologists to comment on the fundamental inadequacy of our medical model with respect to the realities of health and health breakdowns as social events. Morley concludes his introduction to *Culture and Curing* with this analysis:

"Medicine", in the ethnomedical sense, is to be seen as more than the fiat of the Western medical paradigm. The really fundamental *sine qua non* of medicine in both traditional and modern industrial societies is that it is a social phenomenon and can only be fully understood as such. In traditional societies medical knowledge is far more closely integrated with the institutions and all-encompassing cosmology of the society as a whole than is the case in more differentiated industrial societies. (pp. 15–16)

Later in the same volume Una Maclean, discussing the attitudes toward health among the Yoruba of Nigeria, remarks about our own culture:

We have begun to recognize the importance of social and psychological factors both in the occurrence of disease and in the processes of care and cure. We are aware that bad interpersonal relations can make us feel

ill; we realize that the death of a loved relative can for
a time make our own demise more likely; we acknowl-
edge that a patient's return to health can take place more
rapidly in an atmosphere of sympathy and caring. We
have been late in coming to these realizations about the
mutual involvement of mind and body, partly because
the initial successes of modern medicine were built
upon a mechanistic model which either assumed a dichotomy between body and mind or even proceeded on
the assumption that bodily diseases could be managed
virtually without reference to the person experiencing
them.

But to many other people our distinction between
physical and mental illness and our separation of the
individual from his social nexus are meaningless, and
they have not even made a distinction between sickness
and other severe misfortunes. (Maclean, pp. 153–154)

The standard response to such ideas from the defenders of
the medical model is that we have eliminated the magic,
mysticism, and malarky from the understanding and treatment of illness and have developed instead an objective and
universal science with an unparalleled record of success and
effectiveness. This latter claim, by the way, is subject to
some dispute. Thomas McKeown, for example, suggests that
much of the apparent success of the medical model in the
elimination of rampant diseases must in fact be attributed to
concomitant social efforts toward sanitation and cleanliness.
The claim is a powerful one, however, and it must be remem-
bered that the issue here is not which is better or worse,
traditional or modern medicine, but whether the concept
of health includes an inherent social and moral dimension,
a possibility that the medical model emphatically denies.
If, as I am arguing, the moral dimension is indeed logically
necessary, the rational response should be not to throw out

the medical model but to integrate its biological insights into a more satisfying, coherent, and social conception of human health.

Even in the distant past of our own culture health has often been conceived of and discussed in practical terms as having moral and political aspects. Galen, for example, whose medical writings of the second century A.D. were taught as the ultimate authority throughout the Middle Ages, believed that "only a politically free man could devote the proper attention to bodily hygiene and hope to secure health" (Burns, 1976, p. 206). But the biological and mechanical aspects of the Hippocratic tradition won out in the West and through the years successfully purged the magical, religious—and thus moral—elements out of the practice of medicine. René Dubos sums up this development with the obvious pride of someone who is documenting the progressive enlightenment of his own tradition:

> The fundamental philosophy of Hippocratic medicine is that diseases are not caused by capricious gods or irrational forces, as primitive people are wont to believe. They constitute natural phenomena developing in accordance with natural laws. Disturbances of the body and the mind can therefore be studied just as objectively as any other natural phenomenon; they can be understood by reason and controlled by the wise management of human life. Hippocratic philosophy contends that medicine is not an appendage to religion; it can and should be practiced as true scientific discipline. Commonplace as this attitude appears today, it developed slowly and has yet to be adopted universally. Even partial acceptance of the Hippocratic doctrines has led, nevertheless, to the formulation of a number of principles shaping the theory and practice of modern medicine.

The primary Hippocratic principle is that medicine
should be based on the natural sciences. (Dubos, p. 74)

This passage makes the fundamental issues of our discussion clearer: either health and medical practice are understood as the domain of natural laws, natural science, and
objective truth, or they must be relegated to the domain of
"religion," "capricious gods," and "irrational forces," that is,
things in which "primitive" people believe. Health is either
culturally recognized as a full-fledged moral term, which
means it is virtually useless with respect to the real, practical
needs of human illness and injury, or it is an objective,
technical term that is wonderously effective biologically but
absolutely irrelevant to social and moral concerns. Dubos
reveals the obvious need for the defenders of medical science to drive out the specter of moral entailment still lurking
darkly somewhere around the edges of the concept of health.
    One of the few places where this moral sensibility is still
admitted by established medical authorities and academi-
cians as somewhat relevant is in discussions of the issues subsumed under the term bioethics, an arena that has been
defined as "the critical examination of the moral dimensions
of decision-making in health related contexts and in contexts
involving the biological sciences" (Gorovitz, p. 52). Traditionally included are such topics as euthanasia, abortion,
medical experimentation, eugenics, and definitions of death
and life. In other words, bioethics is the philosophical discipline in which the moral dilemmas faced by doctors are discussed and evaluated. It would be here, then, one would
think, that the deeply embedded moral content of the concept of health would be explored. But in fact, this rarely if
ever happens. Instead, the decision-making processes that
doctors must use and the social values to which they must
appeal are discussed and argued. That is, bioethics normally

reduces to the discussion of professional dilemmas arising from the existence of specialized experts, dilemmas that are morally relevant to the general public but are experienced as true moral concerns only by the medical technicians, and only, it would seem, as an integral part of their normal, and therefore tacitly approved, professional role and functions. Bioethics addresses the moral issues raised by the notion of health only insofar as it recognizes that doctors routinely and increasingly make decisions that morally affect the rest of us—but in which we have virtually no participation and, further, in which we have essentially no rational access or appeal to any participation. As a philosophical endeavor, bioethics takes both medical science and the doctor's role for granted and focuses on the resulting ethical issues that often arise. As a consequence, it is a field of ethics that has virtually no political or institutional content and the moral conclusions of which have almost no practical relevance. Dr. Larry Churchill of the University of North Carolina sums up the field nicely. After quoting a number of practitioners of bioethics with regard to the "rigor and arduousness of ethical decision making," he continues:

> The thrust of these claims for the "hardness" of ethical reasoning is noteworthy. Because of their prominence and force, these claims have the effect of diminishing the importance of moral perspectives which are incapable of full, lucid explication and replacing them with a (rather sterile) notion of expertise. Bioethics, as currently understood, tends to professionalize moral dimensions of biomedicine by concentrating almost exclusively on explicit criteria and procedures for decisions. These criteria and procedures, while not claimed as the purview solely of bioethics, frequently become their exclusive domain by default. The image which animates this professionalization of ethics is that of the expert—

immaculate in his conceptual clarity, tough-minded, the
master of expertise. (Churchill, p. 234)

Thus the moral-objective dilemma with respect to the
health concept remains. Tribal societies, anthropologists,
and even the natural usage in our language seem to imply
that health is an inherently moral concern. On the other
hand, doctors, philosophers, and scientists all tell us that it is
a morally neutral, objective, and scientific concern. The
Marxists claim that it is a political concern but offer little
supporting conceptual analysis. Advocates of holistic health
want it to be a concern of the whole individual but not
of social institutions. Finally, the bioethicists recognize the
moral implications of the term but immediately displace
these implications as relevant only to the rarefied and exclusive practice of experts—that is, people who are by definition, with respect to their expertise, removed from and
superior to the normal moral concerns of everyday society—
a philosophical strategy that successfully turns even the apparently moral and social aspects of health into technical and
professional issues.

It would seem, then, that the notion of health is, at the
very least, probably unique and certainly a complex concept.
At this point, the question of the moral content of the notion
of health would have to be judged to be undecided, despite
the obvious contemporary conviction of the medical perspective, if only because it has as yet to be seriously—that is,
analytically and conceptually—discussed. My claim so far is
that the medical version is indeed far from obvious, that
moral implications do inhere in the concept of health, and
that until this fundamental issue is systematically recognized
and argued, we must hold our entire understanding of health
and medicine to be incomplete and tenuous.

CHAPTER FOUR

MENTAL HEALTH
The Adjustable Mind

It may have occurred to the reader by now that I could be forcing a dilemma where none really exists, that much of the ostensible conceptual difficulty can be cleared away by making the obvious distinction between physical health and mental health. The apparent solution to the confusion would be to recognize that physical health is a necessary human good *and* that it is also an essentially technical, physiological concern. Mental health, on the other hand, is clearly recognized as having an inherent social, and thus a moral, dimension. The moral implications of the concept of health, then, can be seen as arising primarily from the cultural and even subjective concerns of mental health, whereas the objective empirical referent for our judgments of health is connected only with the relatively separate and autonomous processes of physical health.

This argument implies that the concept of health has two distinct meanings and that the sets of criteria for defining these meanings are independent of each other. Moreover, and this is the crucial point, it implies that there can be no judgment of health as such other than that based on one of these two sets of independent criteria or on a sum of both judgments. That is, there can be no concept of health that can be used as the basis for a unified judgment about the life and activities of an individual human being. People do not have health as such. They have physical health or mental health or both. No criteria can exist that combine both of these components of health into a single, irreducible, and rigorous concept. For if there were such a concept, if health were greater than the sum of its parts and a direct and unified judgment could be made, then the moral and the empirical aspects of health would be fundamentally intertwined again, and we would be right back in our original dilemma.

The consequence of this argument is that any particular judgment of health—indeed, any unmodified use of the concept of health—instead of having a clear and unambiguous meaning, can have any one of three legitimate, but logically independent, meanings. Either health is used as a sort of abbreviated way of referring to one of the two sets of distinct criteria, so that health in a particular context *really* means physical health (or mental health), as is the case in the earlier quotations from Toulmin, Engelhardt, Dubos, and Illich, or health refers to the simple sum of both sets of criteria, so that it becomes the recognition of the coincidental combination of physical and mental health in some fortunate individual. Since on this view all of these uses are legitimate and meaningful, only the context of any particular usage can help us to determine which meaning is appropriate, so that the concept is fundamentally unclear and ambiguous. Furthermore, since the criteria defining these different usages are necessarily logically independent (or the argument fails to resolve anything), and since the criteria defining one of these usages are assumed to be in large part culturally determined, then these different meanings could in some cases, even in all cases, turn out to be mutually incompatible, even conflicting, so that the concept of health itself may in the final analysis be internally contradictory.

In the following chapter, I intend to show that when the concept of health is interpreted in this way, it is indeed necessarily self-contradictory and that the consequences of this interpretation, which is at the heart of medical science, for our understanding, our health, and our society have been significant, perhaps even calamitous. Also, I shall argue that this interpretation is incorrect, that in spite of what the doctors and philosophers tell us, health is not an ambiguous and contradictory concept but is in fact quite clear and meaningful. Use of the concept includes an evaluation of the physical and mental (perhaps interactional would be more appropriate) aspects of individual life, but the concept itself is based on criteria that unify these aspects into an indivisible conception of human health that is both morally informed and empirically grounded.

Historically, certain purposes of treatment and practical understanding may have made it appropriate and useful to distinguish between physical health and mental health, to imagine conceptually that one set of health-indicating processes and relations can be analyzed more or less autonomously from another. In this sense the distinction is between ideal types, conceptual simplifications that for reasons of analysis have been abstracted by an observer from a given totality. But to say that these abstractions are independent aspects of health is like saying that politics and economics are independent aspects of a society or that mass and energy are independent aspects of uranium or that heads and tails are independent aspects of a coin. The point is that physical and mental health are different ways of looking at the same thing, and although these different ways of looking have their practical and conceptual uses, those uses are for understanding the thing itself—health—a thing that cannot be coherently understood as simply the sum of these two supposedly autonomous parts. The fact that we have in large part committed ourselves conceptually and institutionally to the notion that the independence of these processes is immanent and decisive is once again an indication of the underlying mind-body dualism in Western intellectual and social history and is not a substitute for an analysis and understanding of human health.

To the degree that this distinction is taken for granted, however, the analysis of mental health becomes far more conceptually problematic than the analysis of physical health, for, as we have seen, it is through the notion of mental health that the concept of health must be related to the individual's social activities and thus to the context of moral judgments. By focusing on the realm of mental health, the empirical referent—the physical body—contained in the concept of health has been abstracted away. All that remains, then, is to attempt to analyze the relation between health and social context in terms of the ideas of sanity and normality, concepts that have virtually no empirical referent and that indeed seem definable only in terms of cultural norms and values. But this of course means that the moral implications of the concept of health are made, through the concept of mental health, to refer finally only to other moral concepts, so that any moral judgments concerning health are at bottom cultural and relative. If mental health, or sanity, can only be judged in terms of the same moral concepts by which social and political actions are judged, then judging a particular set of actions as "unhealthy" in the moral, as opposed to the scientific, sense can only mean that from a particular set of values these actions can be evaluated as morally wrong. In this way health as a moral concept is firmly separated from health as an empirical concept, and with respect to its moral use it indeed becomes similar to other moral concepts, such as justice, freedom, and equality. Rawls's dilemma remains: there is no objective referent for any of these concepts; they can only be defined in terms of one another, and the fact-value distinction remains inviolate.

Nevertheless, the notion of mental health still presents a

problem, because the concept of health has a special status as a moral issue in our language and in our lives. As I have been stressing, health is not only a universal good; it is also a more or less objective state of our bodies. Because of this, although we may, under the proper circumstances, have as deep an emotional concern with health as we have with freedom and justice, we understand and share an opinion of health in ways we do not understand and share an opinion of freedom or justice. Thus, even in its heavily diluted version as mental health, the concept of health still carries special moral and social weight. This has two consequences: first, judgments of mental health have the potential to impose particularly meaningful moral criticisms on social institutions and political actions, in the sense that these institutions drive people crazy. Second, like all claims about health, judgments of mental health can easily be characterized as technical and therefore neutral diagnoses, thus making possible the concealing of moral and political actions under the rubric of scientific objectivity. Clearly, any set of vested social interests that has the power to do so—that is, any dominant social class and institutions—will use its weight and influence to direct the conceptualizing and institutionalizing of the criteria for mental health in such a way as to minimize the former possibility and maximize the latter. Whether or not these interests and influences have had a hand in the genesis of our modern conceptions of mental health, those conceptions have been developed in such a way that these requirements have been successfully fulfilled. This result has been achieved by approaching mental health, just as medicine approaches physical health, through the idea of the conceptually autonomous individual; that is, mental health is considered to be a function of an individual adjustment, mental or intentional, to objective processes in much the same sense that physical health is a function of an individual adjustment,

bodily or physiological, to objective processes. (Indeed, it is
almost certainly because of this individual orientation that
we have come to know it as "mental" rather than something
like "interactional" or "communicative" health.) A focus on
the individual diverts most of the potential social criticism
while maximizing the possibility of a technical and objective
interpretation of mental health. Yet, in spite of the obvious
political usefulness of the idea of the autonomous individual
as the sole locus of mental illness, the very relevance of the
concern with mental health seems to demand that it be recognized as an inherently social issue, that an individual's
mental health be recognized as a function of his or her social
and institutional relationships, and that, consequently, moral
and critical evaluations must be involved. But how can a society theoretically recognize the moral and social aspects of
mental health without opening the door to too much moral
and social criticism? It is this dilemma that has made the
notion of mental health so problematic, for, as it turns out,
the distinction between physical and mental health has only
served to displace the essential tension between the technical and moral aspects of the concept of health to another
level, and it is here, with physiology and biology held more
or less in abeyance, that the theorists of mental health must
try to resolve the relation of the mind to social life.

These apparent moral implications have left the therapeutic understanding of mental health less clearly defined and
less generally accepted than the corresponding medical
understanding of physical health. Many conflicting theories
have been offered, each purporting a "scientific" approach.
Certainly the most famous and influential of these approaches
is contained in the theories of Sigmund Freud. Freud was
the first to assert that the issues of mental health and illness
occupy a distinct and separate conceptual realm from those
of physical health, that the understanding and treatment of

mental symptoms require procedures and a vocabulary that
are uniquely psychological, and that understanding and treatment depend upon such things as consciousness, memory,
and social contacts rather than on the organs, cells, and tis-
sues of biology. According to Freud, a fundamental concept
that is "indispensable to us in psychology" is the notion of an
"instinct." Instincts belong to the larger class of stimuli, but
only two kinds of stimuli exist, the instinctual ones and the
physiological ones. "We have now obtained material necessary for discriminating between stimuli of instinctual origin
and the other (physiological) stimuli which operate on our
minds" (Freud, 1957, p. 72). The difference between instinctual and physiological stimuli is that the former originate
within the body while the latter originate outside—the difference between "needs" and perceptions or pains. Using
this distinction, Freud separates the mental and the physical
absolutely with respect to the understanding of mental life:

> By the "source" of an instinct is meant that somatic
> process in an organ or part of the body from which
> there results a stimulus represented in mental life by an
> instinct. We do not know whether this process is regu-
> larly of a chemical nature or whether it may also cor-
> respond with the release of other, e.g., mechanical,
> forces. The study of the sources of instinct is outside
> the scope of psychology; although its source in the body
> is what gives the instinct its distinct and essential char-
> acter, yet in mental life we know it merely by its aims.
> A more exact knowledge of the sources of instinct is not
> strictly necessary for purposes of psychological inves-
> tigation. . . . (Freud, 1957, pp. 74–75)

The instincts that Freud first identified as decisive for all
human psychology are the sexual and the self-preservative
instincts. Later he added the death instinct and argued that

all human activity, mental and physical, could be understood as an eternal struggle between the sum of the first two, which he called Eros, and the latter, which he called Thanatos.

It should be clear that in making the mental-physical separation as he does, Freud takes his definition of instincts, which he offers as objective, out of the morally neutral and acceptably empirical realm of biology and into the culturally involved and morally infused realm of such things as sex and death. In other words, Freud makes his "objective" referents for the study of mental health definable only in terms of the moral understandings of a particular culture. Indeed, as has been repeatedly pointed out, the sexual instinct, the central mechanism for his entire psychology, is "universally" defined in terms of the historically specific and very Victorian notion of the nuclear family and its sexual mores. Moreover, all of Freud's followers, whether they share his particular theories or not, have based their ideas of the determinants of mental health on concepts that have moral and cultural, rather than physiological, referents. In this way, the first systematic conception of mental health was decisively separated from the main tradition of empirical science.

Nonetheless, even from within a particular cultural framework of understanding, the attribution of mental breakdown can conceivably imply a deep critique of social institutions. Once again, however, Freud provides the basic theoretical mechanism through which this possibility can be and largely has been avoided. First of all, as I have argued, the necessary connection between an individual's mental health and the social context of that individual's life is implied by the very notion of mental health. Freud recognizes that connection, and in his discussion of stimuli, he points out that although physiological (external) stimuli are handled effectively by "hereditary muscular movements,"

> those instinctual stimuli which emanate from within
> the organism cannot be dealt with by this mechanism.
> Consequently, they make far higher demands upon the
> nervous system and compel it to complicated and inter-
> dependent activities, which effect such changes in the
> outer world as enable it to offer satisfaction to the inter-
> nal source of stimulation. . . . (Freud, 1957, p. 73)

It is the instinct's relation with the outer world that is problematic and is thus the locus of mental illness. The instinct
even directs the nervous system; that is, an instinct can
pressure the individual to act in such a way as to change the
outer world in order to provide relief.

From these assumptions it is clear that the theorist could
proceed in two fundamentally different directions: toward a
thoroughgoing critique of the outer world, that is, the social
context, on the further assumption that the satisfaction of the
instinct is an essential requirement for health and thus that
the existing social order is a barrier to health; or to a thoroughgoing psycho-physiological critique of the instinct, assuming that the social context is inherently compatible with
and supports normal health. Freud takes the latter route:

> A better term for a stimulus of instinctual origin is a
> "need"; that which does away with this need is "satisfac-
> tion." This can be attained only by a suitable (adequate)
> alteration of the inner source of stimulation. (Freud,
> 1957, p. 72)

The theoretical maneuvers with which Freud followed this
route were brilliant, both for their obvious insight and effectiveness and for their success in blunting social criticism. By
focusing on sex and the family, Freud dramatically localized
the context through which the "outer world" of social interaction impinges on the instincts. Yet sex and the family only

appear to be local issues; in fact, they are intimately intertwined with the entire context of cultural values and social
institutions. To the degree that Freud failed to recognize
this, many of his followers certainly did, and to the degree
that sexual and familial relations are made the central determinants of mental health, a severe critique of social values
and institutions is implied, centering on those of sex and the
family. Indeed, this implication was immediately recognized
in Freud's work, and not only was he denounced for it, but
his implied critique of Victorian values has had a lasting
effect on the legitimacy of those values in our society. This
moral and critical dimension is the lurking danger in the idea
of mental health, and in their own theories Freud's followers
quickly began to mitigate the master's virtually total emphasis on sexual desire.

However, another aspect of Freud's theory has been trans-
mitted essentially intact throughout the tradition he origi-
nated, and it is this conception that has been most successful
in forestalling whatever more damaging political and institutional criticism might have been suggested by his or subsequent analyses of mental health. This theoretical master-
stroke was the conceptual concentration on childhood as the
fundamental locus and origin of all manifestations of mental
illness. "If you like, you may regard the psychoanalytic treatment only as a continued education for the overcoming of
childhood-remnants" (Freud, 1957, pp. 29–30). For Freud,
the absolute importance of the childhood period is due to
the intensity of the sexual development and responses in
that period. The Oedipus complex, the stages of growth, the
id and the superego—all of these central concepts of Freudian theory relate to the sexual experiences of the child. And
all adult breakdowns of mental health, must be understood
and treated as circuitous manifestations of repressed childhood fears and traumas from the distant past.

With the discovery of infantile sexuality and the tracing back of the neurotic symptoms to erotic impulse-components we have arrived at several unexpected formulae for expressing the nature and tendencies of neurotic disease. We see that the individual falls ill when in consequence of outer hindrances or inner lack of adaptability the satisfaction of the erotic needs in the sphere of reality is denied. . . . The flight from the unsatisfying reality . . . takes place over the path of regression, the return to earlier phases of the sexual life. . . . This regression is seemingly a twofold one. . . . Both sorts of regression focus in childhood and have their common point in the production of an infantile condition of sexual life. (Freud, 1957, p. 30)

Though it is obviously insightful, for our purposes here the theoretical emphasis on childhood as the relevant social context for matters of adult health is a clever way of directing attention firmly away from the present political and institutional context of the adult who is suffering mental distress. By locating the problem in the distant past, no analysis of or action on the present social context is called for. Following the logic of this position, the treatment of mental illness requires only removing the purely mental blocks (the repressed memories) from the unconscious of the individual, a task that can be accomplished only through analyst-assisted introspection. In other words, though the problems of mental health are recognized as having inherent social aspects, the understanding and treatment of those problems become, through the displacement to childhood, fully individualized, with only the doctor providing the individually oriented expertise. Thus, mental health, like physical health, becomes a matter concerning autonomous individuals and neutral professionals. The fundamental relevance of the social context regarding issues of health as well as issues of morality is recognized and even integrated into the theory, but then that social context is relegated to a separate and even mythical realm, the realm of childhood, where social interactions are not only long past but are also conceptualized as having a unique and nonrational, a childish, existence, so that no rational, adult actions, and thus no political and institutional criticism, can be applied.

It is a brilliant solution, and Freud goes even further. A sense of guilt is the source of all mental pain, and that guilt exists in all of us as the inevitable consequence of our sexual conflicts as children. But even the best of childhoods (psychoanalytically) cannot help us, as this guilt exists in all of us phylogenetically, that is, as a deeply but unconsciously experienced species-guilt that has been implanted in the unconscious since the killing of the primal father by his sons at the dawn of human history:

> It can also be asserted that when a child reacts to his first great instinctual frustration with excessively strong aggressiveness and with a correspondingly severe superego, he is following a phylogenetic model and is going beyond the response that would be currently justified; for the father of prehistoric times was undoubtedly terrible, and an extreme amount of aggressiveness may be attributed to him. . . . We cannot get away from the assumption that man's sense of guilt springs from the Oedipus complex and was acquired at the killing of the father by the brothers banded together. On that occasion an act of aggression was not suppressed but carried out; but it was the same act of aggression whose suppression in the child is supposed to be the source of his sense of guilt. (Freud, 1961, p. 78)

Thus Freud removes the relevant social context not only to the childish past but also to prehistory, and thus the possibility of acting intelligently and politically on the outer world to make it more compatible with human needs is decisively denied. Freud defines mental health morally, analyzes it scientifically, locates its cause irretrievably in the past, and treats it therapeutically as existing totally in the minds of individuals. Given the assumption of the independence of mental and physical health, and the problems it raises, his is an impressive achievement.

Freud's theoretical maneuver of distancing the therapeutically important social context to the period of childhood has become a standard element of most subsequent psychoanalytic and psychiatric theories, even of those that interpret the importance of that period in very different ways. As Heinz Hartmann put it:

> The genetic approach has become so pervasive, not only in psychopathology but also in psychoanalytic psychology in general, that in analysis phenomena are often grouped together, not according to their descriptive similarities but as belonging together if they have a common genetic root (oral character, anal character). (Hartmann, p. 155)

A good example of the strength and effect of this reliance on the appeal to childhood can be found in the work of Harry Stack Sullivan, a therapist in the Freudian tradition who nevertheless rejects much of Freud's theories and stresses the social, as opposed to the instinctual, development of the individual.

> One sees that there is no *essential* difference between psychotherapeutic achievement and achievements in other forms of education. There is, in each, an alteraction in the cultural-social part of the affected personality, to a state of better adaption to the physio-chemical,

> social, and cultural environment. . . . The principal
> factors responsible for the apparent gap between the
> ordinary good educative techniques and the orthodox
> psychoanalytic procedures are to be found in the pecu-
> liar characteristics of very early experience—*viz.*, that of
> the first 18 to 30 months of extrauterine life. (Sullivan,
> p. 179)

Here even the socially oriented psychoanalyst expresses his
commitment to infancy as the crucial period for mental
health and at the same time reveals the full extent of the
individually centered therapeutic effort. The "affected personality" in its "cultural-social" life must be "better adapted"
to the "social and cultural environment." Even though Sullivan stresses the fundamental importance of social experiences for the understanding of matters of mental health, his
work never suggests that the social context could be or would
ever need to be consciously criticized and acted on in order
to improve the conditions for mental health. The individual
must be "adjusted," not the society; no moral or political
criteria apply to an understanding of the word "better" as he
uses it, for, like the notion of "better physical health," it is a
purely technical usage, only in this case it refers to the "objective" conditions of childhood experiences rather than to
the "objective" conditions of physiological functioning.

Finally, even further from the Freudian tradition, we can
consider a passage from Carl Rogers, an existentialist psychologist and one of the major founders and proponents of
the modern self-oriented humanist psychology.

> This, as we see it, is the basic estrangement in man. He
> has not been true to himself, to his own natural organ-
> ismic valuing of experience, but for the sake of preserv-
> ing the positive regard of others has now come to falsify
> some of the values he experiences and to perceive them

only in terms based upon their value to others. Yet
this has not been a conscious choice, but a natural—
and tragic—development in infancy. The path of development toward psychological maturity, the path of
therapy, is the undoing of this estrangement in man's
functioning, the dissolving of conditions of worth, the
achievement of a self which is congruent with experience, and the restoration of a unified organismic valu-
ing process as the regulator of behavior. (Rogers, p.
220)

Once again infancy is singled out as the inevitable cause, and
the task of the therapist, the job for the doctor, is to "restore
the self" to where it becomes "congruent with experience."
In this case, even the language of physical health and the
medical model is used; only the process referred to is "man's
functioning," rather than "physiological functioning." In the
therapeutic tradition, then, the complete focus on the individual as needing to be helped, as having only internal problems, whatever their sources, is secure.

However, another approach to the issues of mental health
has fundamentally challenged the entire conception of the
psychoanalytic tradition. The approach of behavioral psychology, of operant conditioning, is a theoretical perspective
that stresses its compatibility with experimentation and precise measurements, a demand to which the Freudians never
succumbed. According to this view, there is nothing unique
or independent about the problems of mental health and
illness, and the Freudian assumption that there are special
aspects and entities concerning the mental life, such as the
unconscious, entities that can only be understood through a
special and nonempirical conceptual framework, is simply
mystification and bad science. Psychology must be regarded
as another branch of the empirical science of human behavior
—indeed, one that is finally reducible to biology. In an ar-

ticle titled "What is Psychotic Behavior?" B. F. Skinner, the
major founder and theorist of behavioral psychology, suggests:

> What is needed is an operational definition of terms.
> . . . Thus it might be possible to set up acceptable
> definitions of instincts, needs, emotions, memories,
> psychic energy, and so on, in which each term would
> be carefully related to certain behavioral and environ-
> mental facts. . . . A more reasonable program at this
> stage is to attempt to account for behavior without ap-
> peal to inner explanatory entities. We can do this within
> the accepted framework of biology, gaining thereby not
> only a certain personal reassurance from the prestige of
> a well-developed science, but an extensive set of exper-
> imental practices and dimensional systems. (Skinner, p.
> 290)

With respect to mental illness, Skinner writes: "psychotic behavior, like all behavior, is part of the world of observable
events to which the powerful methods of natural science
apply and to the understanding of which they will prove
adequate" (p. 293).

In the context of the argument I am developing, this is a
particularly interesting position, for by denying the traditional independence of the concept of mental health from
the theories of biology and physiology, Skinner also denies
that the notion of mental health can be used to resolve the
moral dilemma raised by the concept of health itself. In
other words, if the issues of mental health and illness can
really be reduced to the objective processes of empirical
science, what happens to the moral issues raised by the fact
that judgments of mental health are still based upon judgments of social interaction and thus must still be infused
with cultural values?

The answer to this problem is made clear in a paper by Leonard Ullmann and Leonard Krasner, who decide that the concept of mental health is virtually meaningless in the process of reporting that other analysts have found

> that the current definitions were unworkable and at variance with each other. Such findings are not surprising in view of the questionable model on which a concept of "mental health" is based. Definitions of adjustment must be situation specific. . . . The definition of adjustment shifts from time to time and from place to place. (Ullmann and Krasner, p. 298)

The authors feel that the concepts of mental health and mental illness must be replaced by the more meaningful and useful concepts of adaptive and maladaptive behavior.

> Behavior that one culture might consider maladaptive, be it that of the Shaman or the paranoid, is adaptive in another culture if the person so behaving is responding to all the cues present in the situation in a manner likely to lead to his obtaining reinforcement appropriate to his status in that society. Maladaptive behavior is behavior that is considered inappropriate by those key people in a person's life who control reinforcers. (p. 298)

In other words, adaptive and maladaptive behavior—the cultural equivalents of mental health and illness—must be defined culturally. "Normal" behavior in a social setting can only mean what the people in control decide it means. Thus, it is entirely a question of social values, and the use of the concept health, with its implication of more objective standards, is simply inappropriate. With this analysis, the moral connotations of the concerns of mental health, or adaptive behavior, are explicitly recognized and embraced, except that the relevance of the concept of health with respect to these concerns is then rejected, or at least soft-pedaled, as it is by Skinner and other behavioralists, in order to maintain the concept's objective purity. The standards for mental health are effectively relativized. The individual must be adapted or adjusted to whatever social institutions and values happen to be present or imposed. For, with respect to conscious social life, no appeal to a universal and morally necessary criteria for evaluating that life is possible, as it is possible with the concerns of physical life.

From this analysis, it would appear that the evaluation and regulation of "proper" social interaction, proper behavior, should be left to the law, the politicians, and the philosophers rather than to the doctors and scientists, since the latter are established as the protectors of cultural values rather than as the carriers of objective and neutral knowledge. And indeed, this is the position taken by many critics of the practice of psychiatry, notably, as we shall see, by Thomas Szasz. Led by Skinner, however, the behavioralists not only argue that the techniques and theories of behavioral psychology are objective, neutral, and scientific, even biological and physiological, they also argue that these techniques and theories can and should be used in therapeutic situations to establish and maintain mental health, or adaptive behavior, in maladjusted individuals. That is, the specific behavioral goals of such therapy are completely determined by whatever the larger society happens at the moment to accept as "normal," or, more precisely, whatever the rulers and controllers of the society happen to be accepting as "normal." The work of these therapists, like that of medical doctors, is seen as socially neutral, even though the goals to be reached are admittedly cultural and political.

Moreover, the techniques involved are claimed to be empirical and physiological *in the same sense* as those employed to establish physical health; they work not through the consciousness and purposes of the individual but through the autonomous and necessary mechanisms of natural physiological processes. In other words, behavioral psychology, according to the behavioralists, is effective in the same way that antibiotics and surgery are effective: it works independently of an individual's desires or intentions and produces the "proper" behavior strictly through the use of the natural and empirical regularities of the human organism. Maladaptive individuals can be turned into adaptive individuals in the same sense that a stomach can be pumped or a broken arm can be set. The "mental" aspect of mental health has been fully exorcised.

The implications of this theory might well make some of us a bit nervous, for we may not be quite ready to be "adjusted" to the social norm in a scientific way. Yet these possibilities are clearly and proudly articulated throughout the literature of behavioral psychology, or learning theory, as it is sometimes called. Though the emphasis is always on the success of the techniques in "curing" disturbed neurotics and psychotics, some of the examples of experiments conducted to establish the correctness of the theory would seem to indicate that a great deal of nervousness is indeed justified. Hans Eysenck, for example, first establishes his scientific credentials: "I would point out that learning theory is an exact science, which has elaborated quite definite rules about the establishment of conditioned reflexes . . ." (Eysenck, p. 344). Then he states the theoretical approach and its relation to mental health: "modern learning theory . . . would claim that neurotic symptoms are *learned patterns of behavior* which for some reason or other are *unadaptive*" (Eysenck, p.

339, his italics). Mental illness is identified with unadaptive behavior, and neither is given any further definition. However, Eysenck tells a story to illustrate both.

> The paradigm of neurotic symptom formation would be Watson's famous experiment with little Albert, an eleven month old boy who was fond of animals. By a simple process of classical Pavlovian conditioning, Watson created a phobia for white rats in this boy by standing behind him and making a very loud noise by banging an iron bar with a hammer whenever Albert reached for the animal. The rat was the conditioned stimulus in the experiment, the loud fear-producing noise was the unconditioned stimulus. As predicted, the unconditioned response (fear) became conditioned to the C.S. (the rat), and Albert developed a phobia for white rats, and indeed for all furry animals. . . . The fear of the rats thus conditioned is unadaptive (because white rats are not in fact dangerous) and hence is considered to be a neurotic symptom. (p. 339)

Thus, unadaptive behavior is a neurosis by definition, and the symptoms associated with it can be either created or taken away through the proper conditioning. We are not told, however, if little Albert was ever reconditioned to once again be fond of white rats and all furry animals. Only the stimulus is important: "According to learning theory, we are dealing with unadaptive behavior conditioned to certain classes of stimuli; no reference is made to any underlying disorders or complexes in the psyche" (Eysenck, p. 343). And with the proper stimuli and reinforcement, whatever behavior patterns are desired can be instilled without concern for or interference from human consciousness: "Patterns of behaviors are increased, shaped, and maintained through reinforcement" (Ullmann and Krasner, p. 301). In another

example, Eysenck tells us of the cure of some other children's "neuroses":

> As an example of the cure of deficient conditioned re-
> sponses, let me merely mention *enuresis nocturna*,
> where clearly the usual conditioned response of waking
> to the conditioned stimulus of bladder extension has not
> been properly built up. A simple course of training, in
> which a bell rings loudly whenever the child begins to
> urinate, thus activating an electric circuit embedded in
> his bedclothes, soon establishes the previously missing
> connection, and the extremely impressive list of suc-
> cesses achieved with this method . . . speaks strongly
> for the correctness of the theoretical point of view which
> gave rise to this conception. (p. 342)

Thus, by a simple application of electricity, a child may be
"cured" of bedwetting, while the rest of us may be "cured" of
any number of unadaptive behaviors.

As Eysenck sees it, human neurosis is exactly the same as
animal neurosis: studies show that both are "but simple conditioned fear responses of the kind called for by our theory,"
and both can be dealt with directly and effectively by the
proper kind of reconditioning, without involving such things
as consciousness and memories, and certainly without involving moral values. Mental health is the same for humans
as it is for animals, as Skinner tells us explicitly:

> The objection is sometimes raised that research of this
> sort reduces the human subject to the status of a re-
> search animal. . . . Medical research has met this prob-
> lem before and has found an answer which is avail-
> able here. Thanks to the parallel work on animals, it
> has been possible, in some cases at least, to generate
> healthier behavior in men. . . . (Skinner, p. 293)

All the therapist has to do is to "program" humans and their environment, just as they would "program" animals and their environment: "People who are likely to be important in regard to the maintenance of new adaptive behavior can be taught and literally programmed as alternate therapists." With respect to children, "The therapist's goal is to program the parents to respond to and nurture the desired changes toward adaptive behavior" (Ullmann and Krasner, p. 303). But of course the questions remain: Who desires the changes? Who does the programming? Who is defining "adaptive"?

Behavioral psychology denies the conceptual and analytic independence of mental health from physical health while at the same time recognizing that it is inherently a matter of social values in a way that physical health is not. Behavioral theorists try to avoid this dilemma by taking the achievement of adaptive behavior as their absolute goal without ever being clear about what adaptive behavior is. In this way, they treat and refer to adaptive behavior as something equivalent to good physical health, as an objective and neutral goal that all of us can be assumed to desire. Everyone wishes to be well adjusted in the same sense that everyone wishes to be healthy. The techniques of behavioral therapy thus share the virtues of the techniques of medicine: they are empirical and effective, and, as techniques, their effectiveness is independent of the values or histories of the human beings involved.

If this view is accepted, the moral-empirical dilemma of the concept of health has been resolved; both physical and mental health have been reduced to neutral and technical practices. With respect to mental health, the techniques are neutral only with respect to the particular social context established by the dominant social values used to define "adaptive" in a particular case. But this is not a problem, since it is assumed as an objective given that everyone in that social context wishes to be made as compatible with those dominant values as possible, just as it can be assumed that everyone wishes to be made as physically healthy as possible. In any particular society, the dominant values, whatever their source, define absolutely the desired goals and behavior of all individuals, so that no one can reasonably object to being programmed to act in accordance with those values, even if one is unaware of the programming; indeed, if one did object, that could only be evidence that the programming was necessary and that more is needed. In other words, the behavioralist claim to objectivity, together with the resulting resolution of the moral dilemma of health, rests on the assumption that no criteria for moral judgments can possibly exist independently of the dominant social values, that therefore no moral criticism of social institutions can be legitimate, and that any such criticism is an expression of maladaption and mental illness and must be conditioned out of existence for the sake of the individual.

With this assumption the behavioralists establish the particular society of reference as an absolute value, thus objectifying "adaptive behavior." But unfortunately, this assumption denies itself: it is necessarily a moral one, and yet to be meaningful it must be universally true, a possibility that it is intended to disallow. Behavioralists are deeply involved in moral issues even as they are denying the relevance of such issues to their theories and techniques. Their assumption about the objectivity of the dominant social values implies that those values are all of a piece, that no contradictions exist. But this is certainly not the case today and probably has never been true of any human society. The values of our society are constantly in conflict, and any behavioral therapist must select from among competing values the ones he or she will use as a basis for defining and conditioning adaptive behavior, a selection that cannot be made on objective grounds. Also, the analysis of human consciousness, for all its attendant conceptual problems, cannot be so easily dismissed as irrelevant to the scientific understanding of social interaction and individual behavior, for to do so is to declare that human actions and human life can be reduced, as far as science is concerned, to direct observations of stimuli and responses. But since the disagreement is over exactly the question of what human actions are, this declaration can only be a conceptual assumption, not an empirical truth. That is, it can only serve to *define* how human actions are to be observed and understood from this perspective; it cannot be a claim that this is what human actions are in some universally true sense. In this context, the interpretation of human actions leads directly to how human beings will be treated by powerful institutions in a particular society; that is, the defining of "human actions" is an inherently moral concern. As a result, this conceptual declaration is also of necessity an implicit declaration of an underlying moral assumption about the nature of human society and human life. Behavioral theory depends on this moral assumption, as does its claim to an objective treatment of mental health. The theorists try to obfuscate the need for this assumption by claiming that their analysis is neutral with respect to social values. But ultimately, when the arguments are based on a definition of human actions, the position that all societies are equally moral—that is, that morality is not a relevant consideration—requires as much a moral choice as does the position that some societies are more moral than others.

The behavioralists make the choice that, with respect to scientific knowledge, with respect to the "objective" concerns of health and therapy, human beings are just like animals. The obvious implication is that it becomes both reasonable and moral for professionals and experts, and for those who can direct professionals and experts, to treat people like animals with regard to everything from their most political to their most personal activities. I am not arguing that the behavioralist position is mistaken and that therefore the techniques it recommends will not work; indeed, they seem to work quite well. I am only suggesting that it is an inherently value-laden, not an objective, position and that in this sense it is somewhat less than candid. I am also suggesting that although this lack of candor about moral assumptions is shared by most other theories of mental health—indeed, by virtually all theories of social life—the nature of the techniques being developed make it particularly disturbing in this case. Unlike Freudian analysis, behavioral techniques do not assume a conscious subject; that is, they do not depend upon the awareness and participation of the individual. Thus, under the guise of objective science, the behavioralists are striving to develop the ability to program and condition people independently of their conscious interests or resistance. In the fullest practical sense, this is probably not possible (at least, it contradicts my own definition of what human actions and human beings are), but to the degree that it is possible to practice such techniques on a large scale, they would clearly tend to make the people conditioned by them into the kind of beings behavioralism assumes they are. As the behavioralists tell us, people tend to act the way they are treated, and if they are treated like nonconscious animals intensely enough, they will begin to act like nonconscious animals, completely dependent upon external programming. What this means is that the decision about how to treat people is a moral one, not an objective one, and I can imagine that most of us would be morally opposed to the idea of creating a population of programmed, nonconscious people. Yet the behavioralists claim they are not only developing the techniques to do this, they are widely and proudly justifying

these efforts as rational, legitimate, and scientific. They explicitly and consciously offer these techniques to "the key
people who control reinforcers," that is, to the people with
the power to control social institutions.

Significantly, a consequence of the obscuring of the moral
assumption is a theory that denies the importance of the very
basis and uniqueness of human life: the possibility of human
consciousness. Such a theory is promoted as providing scientific knowledge and beneficial technology—as being a contribution to human health. The idea of health is important,
for behavioralism is clearly offered as an effort to resolve the
moral dilemma of health, particularly of mental health. The
model is derived from the sciences of physical health, and,
in the words of Skinner, "A comprehensive set of causal
relations stated with the greatest possible precision is the
best contribution that we, as students of behavior, can make
in the cooperative venture of giving a full account of the
organism as a biological system" (Skinner, p. 290). Here the
real power, as well as the near total misunderstanding, of the
concept of health becomes clear. For Skinner's and his followers' efforts to give mental health a completely empirical
referent, to exorcise the unmistakable but obscure moral
connotations of the "mental entities" of the Freudian tradition, lead them to the seemingly desperate measure of understanding human health as something that can only be
achieved through a theory and techniques that deny the
meaning of human consciousness—that is, human *health* can
only be achieved at the expense of *human* health. The only
other possibility is to accept and theoretically embrace the
moral and social implications of the concept of health, and as
scientists, even as biological and medical scientists, the behavioralists find this possibility completely unacceptable. For
they share with all other theorists and philosophers of health
not only the conviction that health is a morally neutral is-

sue but also the certainty that it is essentially a concern of individuals. Health can only be understood and treated as an empirical problem of individuals, and behavioralism, together with biology, constitutes one of the most rigorous, though finally contradictory and unsettling, efforts in that direction.

But it is not the last, nor even the most unsettling. Following the general empirical and biological perspective of behavioralism, but with a much more direct and even less interactional approach to the treatment of nonnormal behavior or "mental disease," are the surgical and biochemical efforts to understand and control human actions. In these cases the hard "scientific" attitude of behavioralism toward mental life is complete; what have been recognized as issues of consciousness and experience, or even interaction and reinforcement, are reduced to internal, physiological processes. Problems of mental health are identified simply as further problems of physical health, and the study and treatment of mental illness becomes just another branch of medicine. All effort is directed toward understanding the physical processes that can lead to surgical or chemical intervention and cure.

Perhaps the clearest example of this approach is the effort to understand schizophrenia as a physical disease rather than as a vague collection of symptoms involving identity, interaction, and communication. Scientists are trying to locate and isolate a chemical imbalance in the brain that can be identified as the cause of schizophrenia and treated medically, just like any other physical breakdown. Optimistically, this approach could be understood as leading to a recognition that the traditional issues of mental health can only be understood as having to do with both the body and the mind, as revealing the conceptual unity of factors that we now separate as independent aspects of either biology or society.

As Harvard professor of psychiatry Seymour Kety suggests, "Those interested in exploring the biologic aspects of schizophrenic disorders cannot with impunity ignore the psychologic, social, and other environmental factors which operate significantly at various stages of their development" (Kety, p. 99).

In the context of the prevailing idea of health, however, an interest in reconceptualization is not likely; indeed, other instances of a strict biological approach indicate that any such optimism is decidedly misplaced. Perhaps the most overtly gruesome of these interventionist techniques is the practice of psychosurgery—the effort to modify and control disruptive or "ill" behavior through the simple expedient of cutting through or cutting out parts of the brain. This technique has been employed in mental hospitals and prisons, where it is seen as a "cure" for the "sickness" of violence and criminality. Though the extent of this practice is unknown, it is certain that the government, through the now defunct Law Enforcement Assistance Administration, has in the past given many large grants to neurosurgeons to develop and establish the effectiveness of these operations. And the neurosurgeons seem convinced. According to Dr. O. J. Andy, a neurosurgeon at the University of Mississippi Medical Center who has performed lobotomies on "neurotic" adults, "aggressive" adolescents, and "hyperactive" children as young as six:

> There's no question that behavior can be controlled. We have performed surgery on patients in which psychosurgery has been very effective in controlling behavior or resulting in it being altered so that it conformed more with normal human beings in contrast to one that's at the extremes of behavior. . . . Lobotomies have reduced the tension level to a degree compatible with society. . . . These individuals will not be contributors to society, but at least they will be tolerated. (Heath, pp. 8–9)

But what is "normal behavior"? What kind of behavior is "compatible with society"? Since these terms are not objective but can only refer to social values, it generally seems that the people who are considered abnormal or incompatible belong to specific social and economic groups. Dr. Walter Freeman, the author of a textbook called *Psychosurgery* and the performer of four thousand lobotomies, feels that the people best suited for his skills are old people, poor people, people with low skills and low education, and women, particularly black women.

> The operation permitted people to function where little was required of them. Therefore it would be suitable for a woman of whom you expected nothing but that she do a minimal amount of housework; whereas men weren't wanted under those restricted conditions, except occasionally in the very lowest laboring groups. Women have been more easily subjected to abuse; they make better victims; they tend to submit more easily to victimization and they have less power in general. (Heath, p. 10)

As a variation on the surgical procedure, doctors have also been developing techniques for achieving the behavioral effects of lobotomies through implanting electrodes in the brain, a technique that allows the doctor to destroy brain cells in accordance with the observed behavior of the conscious "patient," so that the possibilities of precise control are much improved.

But for all the inadvertent shivers these procedures generate in us, the most accepted, the most widespread, and almost certainly the most potentially effective, as well as the most disturbing, consequences of the biological approach to mental health are the result of the development and use of drugs to modify and control behavior. The general availability of tranquilizing drugs is relatively recent, but they

are now the most heavily prescribed drugs in the United
States, both as a general drug category and as individual
drugs, with diazepam (Valium) being the nation's number
one drug (Hughes and Brewin, p. 9). Most of our institutionalized mental patients, as well as most of the elderly in
nursing homes and many prisoners, are kept constantly se-
dated, drugged into a state of semiactivity and semicon-
sciousness. Indeed, the introduction of tranquilizing drugs
has been hailed as a major breakthrough in the treatment, if
not the understanding, of mental illness, and their use has
brought about a significant increase in the number of mental
patients who can be released from mental institutions. In
1958 Dr. Harold Himwich, director of the Galesberg State
Research Hospital in Illinois, reviewed the state of the art:

> The growing population of our mental hospitals indi-
> cates that advances prior to the advent of new drugs
> were not adequate to cope with the problem of mental
> disease. Much was left to be desired, therefore, from
> the therapeutic viewpoint. Psychoanalysis is a better
> weapon in the management of the neurosis than of the
> psychoses. Electroshock is a comparatively severe pro-
> cedure . . . which greatly benefits patients with depres-
> sion and is of value in the management of excessively
> hyperactive patients to maintain the uneasy status quo
> which characterizes hospitals not using tranquilizing
> drugs. Insulin hypoglycemia appears to be more effec-
> tive than electroshock for certain types of schizophre-
> nia, but requires highly trained physicians and is costly.
> . . . Another method for treating the distraught patient
> is to stupefy or anesthetize him with an adequate dose
> of one of the barbiturate drugs. . . .
>   . . . Though the immediate situation can thus be met,
> it is not necessarily followed by improvement in be-
> havior. With the tranquilizing drugs, however, the pa-

tient is improved without significant interruption of consciousness—a highly desirable goal in the successful therapeutic process. Even if his manic excitement is extreme and if he must be given a correspondingly large dose, which renders him sleepy, he can be easily awakened and in general can go on with his prescribed hospital activities. With the new drugs, more patients have been returned to society from the state hospitals than with any previous therapeutic regime. We therefore seem to be entering a new era in the treatment of mental disease, and it remains to be seen how far this advance will take us. (Himwich, p. 76)

Drug therapy has taken us a long way, but perhaps not always exactly where we might wish to go. As Drs. Milton Silverman and Philip Lee comment in their study of the effects of drugs and the drug industry on our lives:

Although the tranquilizers and related drugs have significantly controlled mental symptoms, they have thus far failed to cure mental illness, and there is a growing apprehension that their frequent use to cushion or camouflage what are simply the normal problems of living may be seriously harming many millions of patients. (Silverman and Lee, p. 13)

It is with respect to these "normal problems of living," problems that are social by definition, that these drugs have had the greatest impact on our understanding and treatment of individual health. These everyday problems of family, work, success, friendships, and the like are being defined, through the use of drugs as problems of mental health—problems that have a biological and individual solution rather than a social and interactional one. Millions of us are being told by our health professionals that it is reasonable and even necessary for us to tranquilize ourselves, that is, to enter a state of less consciousness and more malleability in order to get through the business of each day and remain "healthy." The concept of mental illness is being identified with all possible social responses other than passive and contented acceptance. At the same time, the idea of mental health is being subsumed under biology, even pharmacology, so that mental health, like physical health, is achievable through a pill. Rather than being a special and independent concern that necessitates its own complex theories and specialized training, mental health is becoming a daily medical issue for much of the population, an issue comparable in conceptualization and treatment to physical health.

This approach to mental health is clearly indicated in the advertisements for tranquilizers in the medical journals. One of these, an ad for Serentil that appeared in 1971, shows a mostly hidden and forlorn face looking through a small hole in a bland jigsaw puzzle. Large type proclaims, "FOR THE ANXIETY THAT COMES FROM NOT FITTING IN." Then the ad elaborates in smaller type:

> The newcomer in town that *can't* make friends. The organization man who *can't* adjust to altered status within his company. The woman who *can't* get along with her new daughter-in-law. The executive who *can't* accept retirement.
>
> These common adjustment problems of our society are frequently intolerable for the disordered personality, who often responds with excessive anxiety.
>
> Serentil is suggested for *this* type of patient. Not simply because its tranquilizing action can ease anxiety and tension, but because it benefits personality disorders in general. And because it has not been found habituating. (Concerned Rush Students, p. 30)

Another such ad, this one for Serax, shows a young woman dressed for housework biting her nails nervously and surrounded by, even imprisoned by, the tools of the housewife —a broom, an iron, a mop, a vacuum sweeper, a brush, a wash pail, sponges, a faucet. It reads, "You can't set her free, but you can make her feel less anxious" (Concerned Rush Students, p. 31). It is important to realize that these ads are addressed not to psychiatrists or doctors who have been specially trained to deal with mental health, but to the medical doctors—the internists, surgeons, and general practitioners who in fact write 83 percent of the psychoactive drug prescriptions. In other words, as far as tranquilizers are concerned, mental health has indeed been identified as a physical syndrome, and its diagnosis and treatment has been, almost by default, given over to the medical doctors. As a result, the treatment for this syndrome, the mental disorder of everyday anxiety, consists entirely of using biochemicals to reduce the individual's consciousness of and receptivity to whatever socially induced mental anguish is being suffered. And once again it should be apparent that in most such cases the decision as to when mental suffering is present—that is, when behavior needs to be adjusted—will be left fully to the "professional" judgment, the social values, of the doctor.

A clear instance of the present and potential uses of this drug-induced conception of mental health is the willingness of many primary school authorities, and some parents, to identify "disruptive" behavior on the part of schoolchildren and to "treat" such behavior institutionally with daily doses of tranquilizers. It has been estimated that more than two million schoolchildren are presently being given Ritalin or related drugs for the control of "hyperactivity," and it has also been estimated that most of these children are from minority groups. This type of child behavior is also diagnosed as hyperkinesis, hyperkinetic behavior disorder, minimal brain dysfunction, functional behavior problem, overactivity, cerebral dysfunction, faulty neurological integration, dyslexia, and neurological dysfunction. Significantly, whereas most of these names suggest brain damage or disease, virtually all symptoms are behavioral; there is no evidence of biological or physiological breakdowns that can be said to cause the observed actions. Since the "disease" can only be recognized in everyday behavior, it is important to know what kinds of actions indicate its presence and thus the need for "treatment." According to widely used checklists given to teachers and parents for exactly this purpose, some of the symptoms to watch for are: "fidgets, can't sit still"; "often into things that don't concern him"; "daydreams"; "slow getting ready for school or going to bed"; "doesn't listen to directions"; "looks for thrills and danger"; "shows off, clowns around other children"; "gets wound up, overexcited on trips or treats"; "wets the bed"; "poor coordination, not good in sports." Thus many kinds of everyday behavior, much of it once thought to be normal enough for children and even for adults, is now being redefined as indicating the presence of mental disease (maladaption) as well as the need for physical intervention, in particular for the regular and extended use of tranquilizers. As Sally Williams, president of the Department of School Nurses of the National Education Association, puts it, "These drugs do not simply slow the patient down. They make the brain function better, and as the brain functions better, the child behaves in a more normal pattern . . ." (quoted in Vonder Harr, p. 14).

According to many of our most respected educators, the institutional potential of these drugs for the treatment and control of children is vast. Harold Shane and Jane Grant, both professors of education, suggested in the *National Education Association Journal* in 1969 that by 1979 school faculties would include "biochemical therapist/pharmacists, whose services increase as biochemical therapy and memory improvement chemicals are introduced more widely" (quoted in Vonder Harr, p. 14). T. A. Vonder Harr, from whom most of this information is derived, summarizes the vision of the late James E. Allen, U.S. Commissioner of Education:

> In a 1970 speech to the National School Boards Association, Allen recommended that a computerized diagnostic center be established in each school system "to find out everything possible about the child and his background." With this information, an evaluation of the child within his environment could be made, and appropriate "prescription" prepared by the experts, and the child's future arranged by the professional staff. (Vonder Harr, p. 14)

Together with behavioralism, all of these techniques, from surgery through electrodes to drugs, unquestioningly accept a pervasive, but vague and value-laden, idea of normal individual behavior. In each case the achievement of this social norm requires the use of methods that conceptualize and treat the individual as a set of physical processes. For the sake of better health, such methods uniformly recommend and induce a lessening in conscious control through physical manipulation. On the other hand, the Freudian tradition of psychoanalysis, which requires the achievement of a heightened consciousness of mentally hidden experiences, depends upon equally value-laden assumptions about instincts—what they universally require in the way of social adjustment and how they operate internally to disguise mental illness as social conflicts. In the one case mental health is incorporated into physical health, and the moral problem of the health concept is dissolved into a general and absolute moral acceptance of the prevailing social order. In the other case the analysis and treatment of mental health are established as decisively independent of the processes of physical health, and the moral problem of the health concept is obscured through the claimed objectivity of nonempirical mental entities and their absolute connection with a forgotten and mythical past. Both approaches take the sciences of physical health as empirical givens and try to understand mental health as an additional problem, whether directly related or not. Furthermore, both focus fully on the individual: health is a judgment about individuals, and the treatment of health problems is uniformly seen in terms of the need to adjust the individual to a recognized standard—an empirical standard in the case of physical health and a social standard in the case of mental health. Objectivity is the guiding principle, and it is tacitly assumed that objectivity is possible about individual matters in a way that it is not about social matters. With respect to mental health as it is analyzed from this perspective, individual and social matters are virtually impossible to separate conceptually. But, it is claimed, by collapsing all the relevant and treatable processes of mental health into the individual, whether into the body or the mind, and by maintaining the sciences of physical health as a guiding model, objectivity can be achieved, and the moral dimensions of the concept of health can be set aside.

As we have seen, however, the issue of morality cannot be so easily avoided, and at least one critic of this approach to mental health, Thomas Szasz, has made this point strongly. Szasz attacks the reliance on the model of physical health as conceptually false and deceptive. For him, the ideas of mental health and of mental illness can only make sense metaphorically, for by their very nature health and disease cannot be mental. "Strictly speaking . . . disease and illness can affect only the body. Hence there can be no such thing as mental illness. The term 'mental illness' is a metaphor" (Szasz, 1973, pp. 305–307). Szasz recognizes that the concept of health contains inherent moral connotations and argues from this that although judgments of physical health can be made objectively, judgments of mental health can only be made on the basis of social values:

> The concept of illness, whether bodily or mental, im-
> plies deviation from some clearly defined norm. In the
> case of physical illness the norm is the structural and
> functional integrity of the human body. Thus, although
> the desirability of physical health, as such, is an ethical
> value, what health is can be stated in anatomical and
> physiological terms. What is the norm, deviation from
> which is regarded as mental illness? This question can-
> not easily be answered. But whatever this norm may
> be, we can be certain of only one thing: namely, that it
> must be stated in terms of psychosocial, ethical, and
> legal concepts. (Szasz, 1970, p. 15)

Here Szasz repeats Toulmin's and Engelhardt's arguments that health is both an evaluative term and an objective, so- cially neutral judgment when used with respect to physio- logical functioning. In addition, he analyzes the idea of men- tal health, as I have done, as an inevitably nonobjective, socially biased concept hiding as an objective one. The con- fusion is made possible, he argues, because of the unwar- ranted use of the concept of health. In other words, he recognizes that health has both a moral and an empirical referent, but he concludes that health should therefore be absolutely reserved for judgments about physical processes, for all discussions about mental health are really discussions about politics and social values.

> The practice of mental health education and community
> psychiatry is not medical practice, but moral suasion
> and political coercion. As was pointed out earlier, men-
> tal health and illness are but new words for describing
> moral values. (Szasz, 1970, p. 36)

With regard to how a society should respond to the kind of behavior we now consider to be the manifestation of mental illness—that is, involuntary acts, as opposed to instances of conscious moral and political acts—Szasz has this to say: "if and insofar as it is deemed that 'mental patients' endanger society, society can, and ought to, protect itself from the 'mentally ill' in the same way it does from the 'mentally healthy'—that is by means of the criminal law" (Szasz, 1973, p. 306).

Here, the conceptual and practical problems that entangle the concept of mental health become evident. Neither the analysts of mental health—whether Freudians, behavioralists, or physicians—nor its critics, such as Szasz, interpret the concept in such a way that it can provide grounds for serious social and political criticism in the name of health, the analysts because they consider it to be completely an individual and objective problem, and Szasz because he considers it to be a meaningless problem. By approaching it as an objective medical concern, the analysts introduce the danger of legitimating the right of authorities and experts, whoever they may be, to diagnose anyone who is in some way different or dissatisfied (nonnormal)—from disruptive children and frustrated housewives to criminals and political dissidents—as mentally ill and therefore as subject to "scientific treatment" to make them "compatible with society." Szasz's argument, on the other hand, leads to the equally unsatisfying but perhaps less threatening practice of responding to many whom we would normally and intuitively think of as in fact ill—that is, as out of conscious control and in need of concern and treatment—as conscious criminals who should be locked away rather than helped. Either mental illness is defined by the authorities and treated as an objective problem, or it is not treated at all.

This conceptual bind is unavoidable so long as the idea of

mental health is used to avoid the moral dilemma raised by the concept of health itself. While physical health remains the paradigm and is seen as morally neutral, mental health must also be either morally neutral or morally infused, in which latter case it is not a matter of health at all. In either case, the practical consequences are not inviting. We have seen how the theorists of mental health defend the first alternative by claiming objectivity for each of their various analyses while in fact assigning the legitimation of science to whatever rulers and values happen to be in power. Szasz defends the second alternative, but his arguments also depend upon an assumption of ethical neutrality concerning the understanding and judgments of physical health. Szasz is right, I believe, about the intrinsically moral nature of the concept of mental health, but to the degree that he is right, his efforts to separate physical health and mental health decisively and to retain the empirical and neutral purity of processes of physical health cannot succeed. For his argument about mental health is really an argument that judgments of human actions can only be made in moral and political terms, as opposed to judgments of the "structural and functional integrity of the human body," which can be made in "anatomical and physiological terms." But it is clear from the new insights into genetic structure that all behavioral syndromes, as in the case of "hyperactive" children and schizophrenia, will soon be translatable into physiological and biological terms, so that drugs or surgery or some other physiological techniques will be increasingly available to "treat" any and all aspects of individual actions. As possibilities advance, mental illness will no longer be a metaphor; indeed, mental illness will *become* physical disease. The need for the term "mental illness" may even disappear, as is happening right now with respect to certain kinds of behavior, such as schizophrenia. Yet, whether the actions are interpreted as manifestations of mental illness or physical disease, the judgments made about them, by Szasz's own account, will still be inherently moral and political, and the treatment of those actions will still have moral and political implications. In other words, the moral and political judgments that are hidden behind the claim of objectivity do not lurk within the concept of mental health, as Szasz believes; rather, they lurk within the concept of health itself.

Szasz's attempt, like those of Freud and others, to separate physical health and mental health will not work, because the concept of health itself, as it is applied to human beings, is too strong. It refers to a more fundamental sense of human life and experience than is available either through discussions of biology and physiology or through discussions of consciousness and behavior. For the same reason, it is not possible for the behavioralists and the doctors to reduce the issues of mental health to the concepts and processes of physical health. The concept of mental health, like that of physical health, points in a confused and misleading way to aspects of human life that are integral to an understanding of human health. But this understanding requires a recognition of the central importance of both these concerns, as well as the acceptance of their essential interrelation and unity. Furthermore, it must be recognized, rather than simply dismissed, that health is quite possibly a moral concept with an empirical referent, a possibility with some intriguing moral and political implications, and one that cannot be logically avoided by the doctors' efforts to individualize and internalize all social conflicts or by their willingness to sacrifice individual consciousness for the sake of individual health.

CHAPTER FIVE

THE HUMAN MEANING
OF HEALTH

So far I have argued that doctors, psychologists, and philosophers have significantly and systematically misunderstood the idea of human health. But if the expert opinion about health is conceptually confused, what recourse is there? Assuming that health is a useful and meaningful concept, what do we mean when we talk about health, and how can we find it out? Moreover, assuming that the physiological aspects of health are fairly well established, what, if any, are the social and moral consequences entailed by this concept, and how are they related to physiology?

Health is recognized as an evaluative term, and I have suggested that it has apparent moral implications. Unlike other moral terms, however, it can be at least partially defined through clear, unambiguous, and convincing empirical criteria. If it were accepted as a full-fledged moral term, this empirical referent would pose a serious problem, for it would logically entail that doctors, as well as the rest of us who are in favor of health—that is, who are moral—be committed to endorse and engage in specific social and political actions, actions that could, on empirical grounds, be judged as "healthy," in that they lead to health. Because this situation might prove embarrassing, or because it is simply logically and morally untenable, which has not been proven or even argued, doctors and medical theorists have based their actions and analyses on the assumption that the empirical criteria *completely* define health and that therefore it is a technical

term that can only morally entail technical and self-directed
actions that are socially neutral. I shall argue that this assumption is necessarily false and that health must be accepted as a serious and socially relevant moral term. Then
I shall argue that its grounding in a set of concrete, universally shared empirical criteria—the criteria of physiological
functioning—may indeed make health our most central moral
term, the one that informs our most important and decisive
judgments about the full context of human life and action.

If this argument is correct, then the distinction between
facts and values, so dear to philosophers, will be invalid as it
is commonly presented. The position I defend will be the
one R. M. Hare calls "naturalism," which he summarizes
with this observation:

> If it were possible to start from empirical premises,
> established by ordinary observation and the familiar
> procedures for predicting the future, and from them,
> by the conceptual transformations which philosophy
> discovered, get to substantial moral conclusions, then
> philosophy would really have done something for the
> solution of practical problems. (Hare, 1971, p. 103)

I shall argue that the concept of health does permit such
"conceptual transformations" and that such an analysis will
indeed lead to important solutions to practical problems,
solutions that will be objectively correct whether or not they
will be practically viable within our present political and
economic system. Hare himself believes that any analysis of
this kind is impossible: "the moral concepts being what they
are, no account of them could in principle be given which
would enable one to pass by a logical deduction from empirical or other factual premises to a moral conclusion" (Hare,
1971, p. 103). I maintain that exactly such a deduction is possible and natural through the concept of health and that the

doctors have had to force themselves into serious and apparent contradictions in order to avoid it. Hare would probably reply that health is not really a moral concept at all, in the sense that no "substantial," that is, social and political, conclusions can be derived from it. This is essentially the position of Toulmin, Engelhardt, Szasz, and many other philosophers: health is indeed a universal good, but only a technical one; it is too general, too specific, or both to provide necessary solutions to practical social problems. Philippa Foot clarifies the issues and points to the philosophical unity on the subject when she summarizes the standard position:

> It would not be an exaggeration to say that the whole of moral philosophy, as it is now widely taught, rests on a contrast between statements of fact and evaluations. . . . One man may say that a thing is good because of some fact about it, and another may refuse to take that fact as any evidence at all, for nothing is laid down in the meaning of "good" which connects it with one piece of "evidence" rather than another. (Foot, pp. 110–111)

With some nervousness, I shall maintain, against "the whole of moral philosophy," that health is a good thing because of some empirical facts about it, that no one can refuse to take those facts as evidence, and that the meaning of health *is* connected with specific pieces of evidence. Indeed, Toulmin, Engelhardt, Szasz, and virtually all philosophers who have commented on the question of health support my position. Since health is so generally recognized as a universal human good because of straightforward physical facts, it again seems curious that the whole of moral philosophy has not paid more attention to it. The idea, of course, is that to say something is good is to show approval of it, and approval cannot logically be entailed by any set of facts. But approval of health is entailed by the facts about it, the facts that connect it absolutely with our ability to be human and thus to be able to make moral decisions in the first place. It is obviously possible for someone to take a position of disapproval toward health, but it is not possible to claim this as a position of principle. One may be against health for oneself or for a specific group of others, but such an attitude must remain either an individual idiosyncrasy or a conscious act of moral discrimination; it cannot logically be made into a general moral rule. For health is an essential attribute of human life itself, and to take a principled moral stand against health is to take a principled moral stand against the possibility of taking principled moral stands. The point is, and this is the general point of the present work as well, that there are some empirical facts so intimately connected with the very possibility of human life, and thus of moral consciousness, that it is impossible to separate them from moral concerns. To do so would be to deny that the moral aspects of human life are grounded in a physical reality—a clearly untenable position to which the "whole of moral philosophy" may nevertheless be committed.

Of course, as far as the concept of health is concerned, no one argues that health is not a necessary and universal human good. Thus the discrepancy between the meaning of health and the whole of moral philosophy remains. The only way out is to argue, as Toulmin and others have done and as the moral philosophers might do (since they have ignored the term, it is impossible to know for sure), that health is a special kind of moral term, one that cannot entail the kinds of moral conclusions necessary for specific social and political actions. This is clearly a weak argument to be used in defense of such an honored and decisive position, but what it lacks in logic it makes up for in believability because of its support for and reliance on the similar and socially legitimate position of medical science. Logically, however, it is a retreat from the strong position that facts and values are separate to the weak position that facts are separate from socially relevant values. Since the empirical referent of health is accepted by doctors and philosophers alike, the only real issue involved is whether the meaning of health can be shown to entail specific social responses to significant moral problems. If this can be shown, as I believe it can, the fact-value distinction will presumably have been bridged. At the very least it will become necessary to think of health as not only an important medical and individual concern but also as an important social, political, and moral concern.

In order to argue the unacceptability of the medical and philosophical conception that health has empirical but no socially relevant meanings, I must suggest that another conception is at once available, clear, and correct, and I must make explicit the criteria by which this judgment of correctness is made. In order to do this I shall use, as Hare puts it, the "conceptual transformations" that philosophy has discovered; that is, I shall proceed through an analysis of the meanings inherent in our use of the natural language. The conception of health that I contrast with the medical understanding is the one available to all of us through our ordinary use of the term. It underlies our normal idea of health as a condition of and judgment on our everyday lives and activities. In other words, it is the necessary linguistic conception that makes possible our regular, nonprofessional use of the term as a meaningful part of human communication. We all use the term naturally, most of us without the benefit of advanced medical training, and in order for that use to be meaningful—which it obviously is, since our judgments about being healthy clearly communicate what we intend—we must all share a basic understanding of what health is.

Yet it is possible to make judgments on the basis of that
shared linguistic understanding without ever bringing to
consciousness and making precise the criteria on which the
judgments are made. In the case of health, the shared understanding is so complete that the meaning of the term is
felt by its users to be apparent, and the prestige of science
has been so great that we have simply assumed that the
doctors mean the same thing by it that we do. In general,
however, they do not, and I shall try to show that our everyday idea of health is necessarily in conflict with the medical understanding of it. To do this, I must determine more
exactly just what our ordinary understanding of health is
and what criteria we use to make judgments of "healthy" or
"unhealthy" in everyday usage. Both inquiries necessitate a
careful inspection of the ways in which we attribute health
meaningfully; that is, I must treat all of us as authorities
because, presumably, we all share the same basic conception.

It could be objected, of course, that even if there are
two conceptions and even if they are in conflict, it makes
no difference, since doctors and scientists are clearly the
authorities. The everyday linguistic conception would thus
simply be in need of correction. Certainly the admission
of two conceptions would not mean that the everyday idea
should take precedence and that the medical idea is wrong.
At least three responses are relevant to this objection, all of
them variations of the obvious fact that health and healthy,
like any other concepts, are necessarily defined by the ways
in which they are meaningfully used rather than by this or
that effort to legislate a definition. It follows that if these
concepts are used more broadly in everyday speech than
they are in their medical versions, then the medical com-
ponent of the conception cannot comprise the complete,
perhaps not even the primary, interpretation. The first re-

sponse is that doctors can be the final authorities on health only if the medical version is accepted; in this respect the objection is circular. Second, if the medical conception is the correct one, then health becomes a technical term, like nuclear fission or photosynthesis, a condition or process that only technical manipulations, either by doctors or individuals, can maximize. This interpretation would in effect deny the moral content that is necessarily a part of the meaning of the term. I believe we have come very close, perhaps as close as possible, to denying this moral content in our almost total homage to the professional foreclosure of the concept. The moral content is there nonetheless, and it constantly reminds us, in nervous and uncertain ways, that there is a felt gap between our doctors' and our own intuitive sense of our health. The same rational hesitancy we feel about giving up our understanding of freedom to the politicians and corporation managers, or our notion of justice to the police, we also feel about giving up our natural and nontechnical sense of health to the doctors. So long as its moral content remains, health cannot be a technical concept. Third, the primary importance of the everyday conception is recognized even by doctors and philosophers, for they do not attempt to correct or replace the way the term is ordinarily understood; rather, they assume that their usage of the term is the same as everyone else's, only more precise. That is, whether they speak to us as patients, to each other, or to their friends and family, doctors, just like the rest of us, use the everyday concept of health as though it corresponded exactly to what they as doctors happen to be experts about. They necessarily legitimate their own idea of health by claiming, fairly successfully, to be experts about what all of us understand and want, thus at once achieving their desired status and confusing us about what health in fact is. If the everyday conception is different from the medical definition, as I claim, then it is necessarily the fundamental standard by which we understand and make judgments about health.

Looking, then, at the ways in which we normally use the terms health or healthy, the first thing that seems clear is that a judgment of health cannot be simply a matter of physical functioning; it must include a reference to some standard of communicative performance and social participation. This would seem to be apparent from the fact that it is possible to judge as healthy someone who is severely physically crippled, though it is not possible to make a similar judgment about someone who is severely mentally or socially crippled. Throughout this discussion I shall refer only to those attributions of health that are direct and ingenuous, tinged neither with humorous nor sad irony. When the television program "60 Minutes" documented the activities and history of Max Cleland, who served as director of the Veterans Administration during the Carter administration and who had lost both legs and one arm in the Vietnam War, he was filmed doing push-ups from his wheelchair, driving a car, encouraging other handicapped veterans, and generally running the VA more successfully than it had been run in years. The point of the program, persuasively made, was that this man would have to be judged as healthy, perhaps as more healthy than many people who are not handicapped. This point was reinforced in a much more critical, even negative, interpretation of Cleland's administrative efforts in *Rolling Stone*. Writer William Woods commented: "His eyes hold the fire which took his arms and legs, and the reports that visitors are unaware of his handicap—claims I had dismissed as pious—turned out to be literally true: he fills a room 'til there's no room for his losses" (Woods, p. 29). The same could probably be said for many other handicapped persons. In these cases health cannot simply be a judgment of relative physical functioning. On the other hand, we would almost certainly not describe as healthy a person in excellent physical condition who had become catatonic, paranoid schizophrenic, or otherwise severely socially and mentally incompetent. With respect to a blind, paralyzed, or crippled person, we might initially doubt the applicability, even the good taste, of the characterization healthy, but with sufficient information and evidence, we could be willing to apply it in good faith and without irony. In this case it would probably also carry the atypical meaning of "remarkable." With respect to obvious social or mental incompetence, however, no amount of evidence of physical functioning could make the naive judgment of "healthy" appropriate. In other words, a severe physical handicap may be presumptive, but not conclusive, grounds for withholding the judgment of health, but a severe and unambiguous social incapacity (assuming such a thing exists, which seems reasonable) is necessarily decisive. It is true that, after a physical checkup, a physician may announce that a catatonic, say, is in "good health," but he would most likely qualify this judgment with the adjective "physical." In any case, physicians are the only ones who would use the term in this technical sense, and that of course is my point.

It follows that the normal, nonmedical attribution of health necessarily includes some inherent standards of at least minimum social competence. When we naively judge someone as healthy, we are commenting to some degree on that person's ability to function in a normal social situation. This is not the quality usually indicated by the concept of mental health; we would not call someone healthy who was fully alert and rational mentally but who was completely paralyzed, confined to an iron lung, or bedridden. The judgment "being healthy" implies some minimum, but not necessarily maximum, combination of physical functioning and social participation. The healthy person must be able in some

degree to communicate and interact with other people in
such a way that the communication itself does not become
severely problematic, and that person must be able to maneuver enough physically so that participation in social interactions does not severely disrupt the more or less normal continuity of daily life. In other words, people who are
healthy are recognized as having a basic responsibility for
both their ideas and their actions. They must have and must
exhibit an essential control over both the substance of and
the relationship between what they think and what they do,
enough control so that the regular activities of social life can
include them and continue without fundamental distortion.
Just what this "basic responsibility" or "essential control"
consists of and how it is determined is a problem to which I
shall return in a moment. For now it should be clear that a
minimum evaluation of social competence is necessarily included in every ordinary judgment of health. An evaluation
of physical functioning is also included and is fundamental,
but the judgment itself cannot be made solely on this evaluation, nor can the evaluation be based solely on technical and
physiological criteria of the integrity of bodily mechanisms.
These mechanisms are important, even essential, and to that
degree the doctors are right: there is an empirical referent
for the concept of health. But the primary significance of
these mechanisms for the judgment of health as it is naturally understood and used is in their social, not their physiological, consequences.

It could be objected here that lay people may, like the
doctors, use the term health in two (or more) different
senses: although we indeed sometimes include social competence, we sometimes intend to use the term in a strict
physiological sense, as when, for example, we see a baby girl
for the first time and remark to her mother how healthy she
is, referring only to her energetic activity and rosy cheeks.

But this objection cannot be correct. First of all, it would make the term meaningless, in the sense that no one could be sure what was meant by the judgment. Second, it is clear that when we use the term even in this case, we are still necessarily referring to the social aspects of health, for we could see the same child in the same physical condition cutting off her little brother's fingers with an axe or setting her playmates on fire and we would not call her healthy. We never see people just as bodies, but always as social actors; therefore, we never judge them strictly in terms of their technical condition. Even doctors must take social values and expectations into account in judgments of health, for it is easy to imagine what a doctor would say of a man who was in perfect health physically but who was constantly trying to cover the office, as well as the doctor and the staff, with red and green paint from spray cans. The doctor's judgment depends far more than is normally admitted on the patient's playing the patient role during the medical procedures. Indeed this has been the point of many recent studies on doctor-patient interaction, studies which indicate how tacit social judgments by doctors severely direct and systematically distort medical practice, particularly with respect to the poor, racial minorities, and women.

The part that personal responsibility with respect to a social group plays in the judgment of an individual's health can be more clearly understood if we consider the legal attitude toward these matters. Even when a defendant's commission of a crime is clear, his or her fate in a legal proceeding can still depend upon the determination of legal responsibility. If lack of responsibility can be established, the defendant will be found innocent of the crime but guilty of a mental breakdown or disorder and will thus be remanded to a doctor's care. That is, he or she will be found to be, or to have been, unhealthy. On the other hand, to be found re-

sponsible is to be judged guilty, not healthy; one can be
dying of cancer and still be guilty of a crime. Thus the attribution of responsibility is a necessary, but not a sufficient,
condition for the judgment of good health.

This example also demonstrates the logical priority and
necessity of the everyday conception of health, since our
basic social institutions rely upon this conception and not the
medical one. It is true, of course, that this interpretation of
responsibility is not common to all legal systems, that many
do not distinguish between actual commission and legal guilt.
But where the judgment of health has not been recognized
as legally relevant to the determination of guilt, it does not
mean that the society has accepted a different conception of
health. We incorporate the notion of legal responsibility because as a society we have accepted the idea that all human
actions are not necessarily moral actions, an idea associated
with the rise of science and the dismantling of an all-per-
vasive religious consciousness. Indeed, we use the concept
of health as one way to formalize and legitimate this distinction. But try as we may to treat some actions as essentially
nonmoral, we must still recognize, intuitively and legally,
that the evaluation of health is inevitably a moral and social
judgment and thus one that both can and must finally be
made by nonspecialists, that is, by judges and jurors rather
than by doctors and scientists.

The standards for attributing responsibility in the judgment of health are closely connected with the recognition of
intention—the quality of human actions that is perhaps most
specifically and uniquely human. Because we communicate
linguistically, because we have consciousness and thus can
think without acting, can make plans, it is possible to separate human intentions conceptually from human actions. This
distinction underlies the legal consideration of health as a factor in deciding guilt. The importance of intention in decid-

ing responsibility, and thus health, can be seen by considering how in certain cases the discovery of intention can completely reverse our judgment of someone's health. Suppose we hear that a man with no physical malfunctions has done three hundred push-ups and is still going. If asked, we would probably decide that he was healthy. But if we then discovered that he had consciously chosen to do those push-ups on the main railroad track where the express was due any moment, we would probably change our opinion and decide that he was sick. Similarly, running thirty miles could reasonably be considered presumptive evidence of good health, but discovering that the purpose of such a run was to arrive at the exact site and time of a nuclear weapons test would be considered presumptive evidence of unhealth. The intentions of an individual, as far as we know them, are matter-of-factly taken into account in our ordinary judgments of that individual's health. When we do not know intentions, we simply assume, in the absence of contrary evidence and without conscious effort, that whatever they are, they are more or less normal and reasonable.

But what does this mean? How are we to understand what people recognize as being "more or less normal and reasonable"? Clearly, reasonableness can be determined only in particular cases on the basis of available cultural values: among some people putting a ring in your nose could be considered healthy, whereas among others it might be considered a sign of derangement. In the example above, if the athlete doing push-ups in front of the train just happened to be exercising during a mass action of civil disobedience as a protest against some policy, such as occurred during the Vietnam War, those who agreed with or understood the reasons behind the action would probably not consider the push-ups as a sign of ill health, whereas others might decide that all the protesters were sick.

The point is that cultural and personal values necessarily enter into every particular judgment of health, so that in this sense many of us inevitably define and use the concept differently. But it is also clear that if we abstract beyond the particular differences in values, we find a more formal element intrinsic in all judgments of good health, whatever the culture. This is the element of rational intention, the determination that an individual's actions or attitudes have been consciously and rationally *chosen* as a response to this particular situation—a response that is manifestly based on values or principles that can be expounded to and understood by others. In other words, the judgment of good health depends pivotally upon the recognition of a directed purposiveness generated by a coherent conceptual framework of conscious choices. This recognition that an action, however objectively futile it may be, is consciously intended and based on a coherent understanding, an understanding we may or may not share, makes us change our evaluation that the action is purposeless, and therefore a sign of derangement, to a decision that it reveals at least the basic ingredients of healthy behavior. It is also this recognition of coherent intention that makes us decide legally that a perpetrator is a criminal rather than a victim of bad health (mental breakdown).

Yet this is what it means to be a human being, to be able to conceptualize, to make choices, to set and work toward goals, as opposed to being in the grip of instinct or reflexes, to be under hypnosis, to be programmed, to be out of conscious control, and generally to have no rational or conceptual choice over one's actions. In other words, the judgment of health as it is applied to individuals in the natural language inherently involves recognition and evaluation of an individual's ability to be fully human—to act and think as a conscious and purposeful human being. When this ability is clearly missing (and there will probably always be confusion on the borderlines), the judgment of good health is withheld, no matter what particular context of values is involved. And of course the ability to make *conscious* choices is the same thing as the need to make *moral* choices, for it is the possibility of moral rules (values) as a guide for human actions and the recognition of moral responsibility as the essence of human action that underlies all of social order and social life. Thus, since the most fundamental criteria for the judgment of health is perhaps the recognition of moral responsibility, health is necessarily and inherently a moral concept. Like freedom and justice, the concept of health, when it is applied to human beings, is meaningful only as a property or quality of conscious and moral actors that distinguishes between the desirable, or fully human, life and the undesirable, or less than human, life. To give doctors and philosophers their due, it is not so much that their criteria of physiological functioning as the basis of health is wrong, but rather that it is incomplete. The notion of human, or moral, functioning must be included as the fundamental element of human health, the element that makes physiological functioning meaningful.

Yet health, as we use it normally to apply to individuals, means even more: it includes a judgment about a person's future and the person's ability to act on that future, both morally and physically, in an effective manner, that is, with essential control. For example, we would not consider someone healthy who had terminal cancer, even though at a particular stage of the disease he or she might be able to carry on daily activities more efficiently than, say, a paraplegic or an amputee. On the other hand, we can and do refer to people with some cases of hemophilia, epilepsy, heart disease, and diabetes to be healthy. We would not, of course, apply the term healthy to the hemophiliac who is bleeding or the epileptic having a seizure or the heart patient suffering an attack, but neither would we consider the otherwise healthy person to be healthy when he or she has the flu or is recovering from an accident. Simply knowing that someone has a disease, even an incurable and potentially life-threatening disease, is not a sufficient reason for considering that person generally unhealthy unless our knowledge of the disease includes the fact that it will inevitably and progressively take over, disrupt, and unnaturally end life. People with hemophilia or heart disease may have to lead somewhat restricted and more careful lives, and the unaffected judgment of healthiness in such a case may also, as with the amputee, imply an additional sense of being "remarkable"; nevertheless, it is a possible and not uncommon judgment. (The feeling that such people are remarkable clearly means that it is considered unusual that with their physical handicaps they can still be active and morally responsible social participants.) The decisive element, then, seems to be our understanding of whether a disease can be controlled so that the individual can be expected to continue a more or less normal life, or whether the disease has taken essential control of the individual's future, so that he or she has already lost the options and potential available in a healthy human life. Thus, an important aspect of the judgment of health is a determination of the degree of control that a person has over his or her life, not only as a conscious and moral actor in the present but also in the sense of being able to choose, subject only to normal uncertainties and limitations, the course of his or her future. Perhaps even more than the notion of responsibility, this notion of control seems to be central to our concept of health, for it includes not only control over our conscious choices (moral responsibility) but also control over our physical activities now and in the future.

Health is a judgment about the full potential of human life as it is understood naturally and meaningfully as the underlying basis—as the precondition, as Toulmin puts it—for any particular content of cultural values. Thus it is both a moral and a social term. When applied to individuals, it is a judgment about their ability to live fully moral and social lives. But what does this mean? How do we judge the content of a "fully moral and social life" other than in terms of cultural values? What are, if any, the real social and political implications of the concept of health? To answer this question, we must look at how the judgment of health is applied to aspects of social life other than individual human performance.

CHAPTER SIX

SOCIAL HEALTH
The Evaluation of Institutions

When we judge other living things, such as animals and plants, as healthy or not, we make these judgments primarily on the basis of physiology and biology, without the necessity of the conceptual and moral connotations we apply to humans. In this sense our evaluation of animal and plant health is similar to the doctors' evaluation of human health: it is based on a set of physical and empirical observations that can be more or less objectively measured. It is probably from this similarity that the medical idea of health is derived: a human is regarded as just another animal or organism with respect to the determinants and judgment of health. But in view of the preceding discussion it would seem that in our normal usage we judge humans and animals with respect to our understanding of their fullest potential. For humans, that judgment involves an additional moral and conceptual dimension.

But what happens when we comment that someone has a healthy garden or has set up a healthy game preserve? Here we begin to consider the concept of health as it can be used to evaluate something that is not a single organism. How are we to understand such a usage? In these cases it seems clear that we are evaluating the overall health of the plants in the garden and the animals in the preserve and that these evaluations depend finally on our judgments of the health of the individual plants and animals. That is, if all the plants or all the animals are healthy (within the natural limits of life span, food limitations, and the like), we judge the garden or the preserve as healthy, but if a significant number are unhealthy, particularly if they are systemically unhealthy, then we judge the garden or preserve as unhealthy. It would seem, then, that the judgment of the health of an interrelated group of organisms would be the sum of the judgments of the health of the organisms themselves and that, consequently, the judgment of the organization or the system through which the organisms relate would be the judgment of how well that organization or system contributes to the health of the particular plants or animals that compose it.

The same point could be made of such evaluations as "a healthy attitude," "a healthy diet," "a healthy relationship," "a healthy environment," and so on. In these cases the term healthy is applied to immaterial, inert, abstract things that are neither organisms nor collections of organisms. Yet the usage is perfectly understandable, and the term is clearly meant as a positive evaluation of the contribution of these things to an individual's health. In all of these cases—gardens and preserves, as well as attitudes and relationships—a clear and meaningful judgment of health is made about many aspects and processes of life other than living individual beings, yet the clarity of the meaning always rests upon an implied evaluation of the health of the individual beings involved. Thus, although health in the normal usage is not just a property or quality of organisms, it would seem from the instances we have considered that any of its more abstract and general applications inevitably refers to the apparent and naturally understood health of those individual organisms, whether human, plant, or animal.

But now consider such descriptions as "a healthy society," "a healthy economy," "a healthy city," "a healthy business." Once again these usages are so widely accepted that they appear regularly in the headlines and articles of our newspapers and journals. A bold headline in the *Los Angeles Times*, for example, announced, "2 Indicators Point to a Healthy Economy," and it was followed by a lead sentence that read in part, "Personal income showed a healthy increase in November. . . ." In another edition the business section included the headline "Healthy Again, MAI Takes a Big Gamble," and the theater section featured an article entitled, "Highlights of a Healthy Season." Finally, an issue of *Newsweek* magazine asserted that "Houston is blooming with health." How are we to understand these evaluations? Clearly, the *Los Angeles Times* was not claiming that the people subject to our economy, or the people working for Management Assistance Inc., or the people involved in the theater season are healthy in the sense that the plants in a healthy garden are healthy. Nothing in the articles refers to the health of these people. Indeed, it is often pointed out, by the *Los Angeles Times* and others, that the people of America, especially some specific groups, are not generally very healthy, at least not by the standards of health that apply to many Americans and that would seem to be compatible with our significant resources of wealth, knowledge, and technology.

At this point I shall digress from the main argument for a moment in order to review quickly some of the data that bear on it. Judgments such as "a healthy economy," "a healthy business," and "a healthy society" necessarily raise the question of the quality of the health of the individual members or participants in the groups or structures being judged. Because I argue in part that in American society in general and in many of its institutions and subgroups in particular there is a significant degradation of individual health, certainly in relative and in many cases in absolute terms, I shall briefly offer some examples of the research and figures on the health conditions of Americans. Unfortunately, such examples are primarily statistical and therefore fail to capture the intense pain and suffering in which many Americans live.

According to the United Nations Demographic Yearbook for 1974, the United States is nineteenth among the countries studied in terms of life expectancy for males, ninth in terms of life expectancy for females, and fifteenth in terms of infant mortality rates. With respect to the last measure, generally considered the most reliable, the United States has been losing its position in the rankings over the last twenty-five years as other countries have successfully lowered their infant mortality rates. The same is true of maternal mortality rates, in which the United States ranked first in 1950 and at least tenth in 1971.

Turning to the more revealing internal comparisons, we can look first at the health consequences of the widespread poverty in this richest of all nations. According to Dr. Geiger of the Tufts Comprehensive Community Health Action Program:

> The health of the poor in the United States—and the health services available to populations in poverty—represents a major, ongoing national disaster, a part of the special human disaster that is extreme poverty in an affluent society. . . . The poor are likelier to be sick. The sick are likelier to be poor. Without intervention, the poor get sicker and the sick get poorer. (Quoted in Hurley, p. 129)

Differing health rates based on race can generally be said to reflect the effects of poverty. In 1974 the infant mortality rate among white infants in the United States was 14.8 deaths in the first year of life per 1,000 live births; among nonwhite infants it was 24.9. The lowest rate for a geographic area of the general population was 11.3 in a "health service area" of Massachusetts, and the highest was 27.1 somewhere in South Carolina. A study of 19 large cities from 1969 to 1971 "showed that whites living in poverty areas had an infant mortality rate almost 50 percent higher than that of whites living in nonpoverty areas, and the blacks, while having a higher rate than whites in either type of area, also have a far higher infant mortality rate in poor areas than in nonpoor areas." Moreover, according to a measure of preventable deaths of infants, "the probably preventable deaths in poor areas were over 100 percent higher than those in the non-poor areas rather than 'merely' 50 percent higher" (Sidel and Sidel, pp. 17–18). Roger Hurley adds that the infant death rate among Indians is 60 percent higher than the national average. He goes on to note that in 1964 East and Central Harlem, with 24 percent of Manhattan's population, accounted for 40 percent of its deaths by tuberculosis, while Bedford-Stuyvesant, with 9 percent of Brooklyn's population, accounted for 24 percent of its tuberculosis deaths. According to a study done at UCLA and quoted by Hurley,

> the Watts area contained only 17 percent of the city's population, but in category after category it harbored nearly 50 percent of the city's ills. It had 48.5 percent of amoebic infections, 42 percent of food poisoning, 44.8 percent of whooping cough, 39 percent of epilepsy, 42.8 percent of rheumatic fever, 44.6 percent of dysentery, 46 percent of venereal disease, 36 percent of meningitis, and 65 percent of reported tuberculin reactors. The death rate in Watts was 22.3 percent higher than for the remainder of the city. (Hurley, p. 134)

The poor in rural areas may be no better off, according to a *New York Times* description of the living conditions of migrant workers on some New Jersey farms:

Many children have distended navels, indicating malnutrition, and many also are ridden with lice and ticks.
Worm-infested infants, left unattended in the camps for
hours by their mothers in the fields, are sometimes
bitten by rats. (Quoted by Hurley, p. 150)

With respect to nutrition, according to Sidels,

some 20 percent of the people in the United States—
particularly among the poor and the elderly—have inadequate amounts or types of food to meet their bodily
needs. It has been estimated that 26 million Americans
cannot afford an adequate diet and that, in 1973, when
the report was prepared, almost half of them received
no help whatever from any federal food program. (Sidel
and Sidel, p. 26)

In the Ten State Nutrition Survey compiled in 1970 by the
Department of Health, Education, and Welfare (HEW) Dr.
Raymond Wheeler reported the following conditions:

The rate of anemia in Louisiana was eight times that of
Honduras . . . levels of growth retardation among low-
income Americans were similar to those in problem
areas of Africa, Asia, and Latin America. One-third of
the children examined up to six years of age showed
evidence of retarded growth. Nutrition deficiency diseases supposedly eradicated years ago appeared in the
survey. The study revealed numerous cases of rickets, a
disease due to the lack of vitamin D found in fortified
milk, and goiter, a disease easily prevented by iodized
salt. (Quoted in Greenstein, p. 311)

In the same year Captain Terrance Goggin, reporting to the
United States Senate on his experiences while conducting a

study for the government of hunger and federal food pro-
grams, gave the following account:

> I was emotionally stunned in going from household to
> household seeing children staring at walls with poten-
> tially tremendous energy but because they weren't get-
> ting food they were like zombies. . . . I was stunned by
> the experience of driving in a White House limousine
> to an airport, going on a plane that was air-conditioned,
> in tremendous luxury, landing in Mississippi, Missouri,
> or California and going off in a car to a shack where
> children, in my opinion, were literally dying, their
> minds were dying. (Quoted in Taylor, p. 93)

The workplace is another major cause of death and illness
in our society. HEW tells us that 14,000 workers are killed
each year in accidents, 2.2 million are disabled, and 500,000
are reported as having developed occupational diseases. In
addition, the Department of Labor estimates that at least
25 million deaths and serious injuries go unreported and
uncounted each year. These figures indicate only the occupational deaths and illnesses already apparent; they cannot
tell us the number of long-term cancers, lung diseases, and
cases of radiation sickness that workers are contracting now,
owing to the vast number of new chemicals and processes
being introduced. Some experts indeed feel that an epidemic of industrial and environmental cancers and other diseases is being generated by industrial conditions at the present time. Perhaps an epidemic already exists. Over 100,000
mine workers now suffer from black lung, a disease that
kills 4,000 each year. Moreover, the coal mining industry
also has the highest industrial accident and death rate in the
United States. About 17,000 textile workers, including up to
90 percent of those engaged in the initial processing of the
fibers, suffer from brown lung, an equally painful, disabling,

and killing disease caused by inhaling the dust associated with cotton, flax, and hemp. Of the 500,000 people who at one time or another have worked in asbestos manufacturing plants, one expert estimates about 35,000 will die of asbestosis, a lung disease, and about 135,000 of lung, chest, or abdominal cancers, a cancer rate three times that of the general population. Another 3.5 million people work with asbestos in the construction and demolition industries. Of 6,000 Western uranium workers, 1,100 are expected to die in the next twenty years from lung cancer. (These statistics are from Stellman and Daum, pp. 3, xiii.) Among farm workers, one Food and Drug Administration (FDA) official estimates 80,000 poisonings and 800 deaths occur each year from the use of organophosphate pesticides in the fields, a chemical originally developed by the military as a nerve-destroying weapon for chemical warfare. Other than death, the effects of such poisonings include dizziness, sweating, cramps, headaches, pus-filled sores, bloody urine, muscle spasms in the esophagus, bleeding from the mouth, nose, and eyes, and respiratory arrest (Zwerdling, pp. 95–96).

And the list could go on. In 1970 the Governmental Industrial Hygienists estimated that from 6,000 to 12,000 toxic industrial chemicals were in common use and that 3,000 new ones were being introduced each year. Yet safety standards were available for only 410 and were being developed at the rate of about 100 per year. In 1968 former Surgeon General William Stewart told Congress that 65 percent of industrial workers are exposed to toxic materials or harmful physical conditions, such as excessive noise or vibrations, and that, according to a survey of 1,700 plants, only about 25 percent of the work force was adequately protected. In addition, it is becoming increasingly evident that the conditions of work in America, while generating a significant contribution to our number two killer, cancer, also have a direct relationship with the tension and stress that underlie our number one killer, heart disease, not to mention the psychological damage resulting from conditions of meaningless, mindless, and uncertain work.

Our general environment is also a health hazard. Most experts, including the American Cancer Society, agree that from 80 to 90 percent of all cancers result from contact with environmental pollutants. Air pollution is estimated to kill up to 500 people each year in California alone and is known to cause many serious and disabling diseases among urban dwellers. Much of our drinking water has been found to be heavily contaminated with chemicals, industrial wastes, sewage, nitrates from fertilizer, and even radioactive particles. Out of 969 water systems sampled in 1970, the water quality of 41 percent did not meet U.S. Public Health Service standards, and the Environmental Protection Agency (EPA) has since found many water supplies to be unsafe. Even more contain significant levels of suspected or known chemical carcinogens for which no standards have been set. In 1972 it was estimated that 600,000 children under six years of age in 241 American cities, primarily poor and hungry children in slum and ghetto areas, either had or were in danger of having lead poisoning, primarily from eating sweet-tasting, peeling, lead-based paint. Lead poisoning can cause brain damage, stupor, seizures, and death. Polyvinylchloride not only has caused high increases in cancer rates among the 2.2 million people who work with it directly, but it also affects many of the rest of us indirectly, since much of our food is wrapped and packaged in it. Michael Jacobson, author of *Nutrition Scoreboard,* estimates that "several hundred thousand Americans are dying prematurely every year because of the food they eat" (McCarthy, p. 61). Our food is so riddled with chemicals, fats, and sugars (the food industry adds about 2,500 substances to our food supply) that each of us now eats 6.7 pounds of food additives a year, and many of these additives, as well as the chemicals fed to animals, such as DES and arsenic, and sprayed on plants, such as pesticides, are known to be linked to serious and fatal diseases.

In response to increasing rates of injuries and diseases, the medical establishment has provided much-needed treatment and services, but unfortunately it has also contributed to the problem. Approximately 300,000 Americans are hospitalized each year because of adverse drug reactions, making this one of the ten leading causes of hospitalization in the country. It has also been estimated that as many as 150,000 people die each year as a result of drug reactions. In addition, abundant evidence throughout the medical profession documents numerous cases of unnecessary surgery as well as professional incompetence among doctors. And, even at its best, it is well known that our medical system services the well-to-do far better than it does those who need it most, the poor and the uninsured workers.

In general, then, the health of members of our society could stand a lot of improvement. To be sure, the combination of medicine, sanitation, and technology has eliminated many of the killing diseases and conditions of the past, but it is also true that new, unexpected, and unrecognized problems are arising every day. The significance of the list I have just recounted is that virtually all of these various causes of illness and death are technologically or institutionally avoidable, given our present state of knowledge and wealth. Such problems are not inevitable byproducts of social life or even of industrialization, at least not to this severe degree. In large part, if not entirely, they are the result of our particular institutional and organizational commitments to the building of an industrial society. Poverty as we know it, and the massive discrepancies of health, opportunity, and social value between the wealthy and the poor, could certainly be reduced or eliminated if we chose to reorder fundamentally our economic system and social priorities. Work hazards could be drastically reduced if the interests of industry and management could be as fully directed toward maximizing both production and worker health and involvement as they are now directed toward cutting and avoiding all possible costs and expenses for the sake of maximizing profit and worker control. Similarly, the environment could be cleaned up if industry were willing to absorb the costs necessary or if government were willing to force industry to clean up its own mess. Both air pollution and automobile accidents, for example, could be significantly lowered if the automobile industry were willing to invest in the equipment to make cleaner and safer cars, or if the automobile, oil, and rubber industries did not use their political and economic resources to prevent the development of local and national systems of public transportation, systems that to some degree existed in many parts of the country a few decades ago until they were bought up and dismantled by these same industries in order to guarantee an even greater need for automobiles and their petroleum and rubber accessories. And the medical system could provide much better, less excessive, and more equitable health care if it were organized according to the needs of human health rather than according to the requirements of professional and corporate profit.

Our society is organized, in other words, in such a way that when its institutions work best, they can make many members of society unnecessarily and severely ill. This conflict between the needs of business and the needs of individual health provides the central incentive for such government action and social services as welfare, Medicare, Medicaid, food stamps, and the like, as well as for such government regulation and inspection agencies as the FDA, the EPA, and the Occupational Safety and Health Administration.

Thus, to return to my argument, it would seem that to judge our society, our economy, or even a particular business as being healthy could not be equivalent to claiming that individual participants in the organization being judged are healthy; indeed, it would seem that in many, if not most, cases the health of the organization would entail significant ill health among its members. We are told, in fact, that often the health of a company, even of the economy as a whole, is simply not compatible with actions that would increase the health of workers or of citizens. In May 1977, for example, General Motors, one of our largest and most powerful companies, told the government that it would shut down production, a step that would necessarily disrupt the entire economy, unless the laws governing emission standards for 1978 cars were relaxed. In other words, the government had to choose between the health of the public and the health of the economy. It is clear, then, that judging the health of a state, a society, or any institution or organization that includes human beings as members or participants is different from judging the health of a garden or a game preserve. Whereas the latter judgment entails a clear and corollary judgment concerning the health of the individual organisms involved, on the face of it the former judgment does not.

This divergence of reference of the concept of health in the case of institutions versus individuals is apparent in the common use of the term. On one day the same page of the *San Diego Union* contained both the headline "Tobacco Industry Remains Healthy" and the sentence "According to health officials, someone in the United States dies every minute and a half as a result of smoking" (Feb. 20, 1978, p. A-8). In the midst of telling us how Houston is "blooming with health," *Newsweek* also noted:

> Houston does, of course, have its share of urban problems. Air pollution and traffic congestion are terrible in

> a city so dependent on cars. . . . Another major prob-
> lem is crime. While the nation's crime rate dropped 7
> percent in the first half of this year, Houston suffered
> a 12 percent increase. Police brutality is particularly
> troublesome. . . . the general prosperity is borne by the
> industrial world's traditional losers—menials, the job-
> less, the unschooled poor. Fully a fifth of the state's
> 12.5 million people survive at or below the poverty
> line—among the ten worst such records in the nation.
> (Dec. 12, 1977)

In the *Los Angeles Times,* readers of the financial page were
presented with this question in bold headlines: "Are Ag Co-
ops Overly Healthy?" This is a particularly interesting usage,
because it is difficult to imagine how one could meaningfully
ask if a human being is overly healthy, except perhaps in a
joking way about an adult who is sexually active or a child
who is simply active. Health is not something of which people
can have too much, but it is apparently something of which
businesses, such as agricultural co-ops, can have too much.
This headline is meant to raise a serious question, a question
that can be seriously answered only by reference to a set
of criteria that can be said to transcend the criteria used to
evaluate the health of a business. In this case these transcending criteria are used to decide whether agricultural co-
ops are becoming too monopolistic, that is, too economically
concentrated and too politically powerful. But, of course,
knowing this only sends us to look for the underlying goals
or values according to which these judgments are made.
Finally, we arrive at a set of social values as the basis for
answering the question, social values that would be defended,
presumably, as representing what is good for the people of
the society. In other words, the question probably intended
is: Does the economic health of the co-ops make life too
noticeably unpleasant (unhealthy) for the rest of us, in the

sense of increased food prices, added inflation, undue political influence, and the like? The question of whether the
social values referred to truly represent the needs of the
people, as opposed to the needs, say, of the economy, of
other corporations, of banks, is not really the point. Inherent
in this usage of the concept of health to evaluate institutions
is the recognition that there is another, superior set of criteria according to which this kind of health, even when it is
fully present, can be judged to be unsatisfactory and thus can
be disapproved of, an impossible judgment with respect to
the health of individuals. As a moral judgment, the evaluation of the health of a society or its institutions seems to be
subject to a transcending moral evaluation in a way that the
evaluation of individual human health, the "universal moral
good," is not.

How, then, are we to understand judgments of the health
of institutions, organizations, and systems that include human beings as participants and members? What makes these
judgments different from judgments of groups and organizations of plants and animals and from judgments of other non-
human things, such as attitudes and smiles. For the reasons
just given, the judgment of institutional health cannot be
completely literal, for if it were, the criteria involved would
be the same as the criteria used for all other literal judgments of health, which would seem impossible, since these
judgments directly and consciously contradict the most fundamental sense of individual health. That is, the people making these judgments know that widespread ill health exists
and that much of it is caused by these same "healthy" institutions. Perhaps, then, this usage is metaphorical rather
than literal. That is, with respect to groups or organizations
of people, the attribution of health is only the suggestion of
an analogy rather than a literal comment on human health. If
this were the case, the usage would mean not the appropri-

ateness of the literal criteria but the suggestion of an essential, though abstract, similarity, like the implication of honesty and personal concern when the ads say that a bank is friendly, or the shared quality of being fleeting and insubstantial that is suggested by the idea that "life is but a walking shadow." According to this interpretation, the basic similarity would have to be something like the abstract notion of "functioning properly" with respect to intrinsic needs. Thus, to say that the description of a society as healthy is a metaphor is to claim, first, that the society is functioning properly *as* a society and, second, that the criteria used to make this judgment are categorically different from literal criteria and that the literal criteria can never meaningfully apply.

This interpretation may seem reasonable at first glance, but I do not think it can be correct. First of all, in the examples above the terms health and healthy are used by the *Los Angeles Times* directly and seemingly literally, not as abstract metaphors, and as a common practice newspapers will only rarely use metaphors in bold headlines and then only within inverted commas. Second, and less whimsically, unlike virtually all conceivable metaphors, this usage is not obviously metaphorical. (One would not be too likely to ponder whether life *really* is a walking shadow, or whether two people *really* are in tune.) The criteria that establish what things can literally be described as healthy or unhealthy are not clear; thus, to call this particular usage necessarily metaphorical is to establish those criteria by fiat rather than by analysis. This is generally what doctors tend to do on the basis of their authority as scientists and professionals, and it is a position clearly supportive of the medical concentration on the body and the individual: the social context of life can be evaluated in terms of health only metaphorically; consequently, being health professionals rather than poets, doctors need not be concerned with it. Yet to accept this argument is only to avoid the issue through the authority of legislative command, not to consider it seriously. One thing, however, is clear: a metaphor is defined as a figure of speech that connects one kind of thing or idea with a *distinctly different* kind of thing or idea for the purposes of suggesting an analogy, and in this particular usage of healthy the difference, if any, is very indistinct.

Moreover, and third, this very obscurity, together with the naturalness of the usage, would seem to suggest that this is indeed a literal application, for although it seems quite natural to refer to a healthy economy or a healthy society— things of which living beings are a part—it seems incongruous and therefore humorous and ironic to refer to a healthy television set or a healthy automobile—things that can be evaluated with respect to proper functioning but whose functioning as machines is neutral with respect to human health. The irony would seem to derive from the sense that to attribute health to a machine is to suggest, incorrectly, that the machine is in fact alive. Furthermore, it seems clearly wrong, and only possible through grim humor or excessive cruelty, to refer, with the meaning of proper functioning, to a healthy war, a healthy depression, a healthy epidemic, or a healthy concentration camp—things that can be said to function properly with respect to their own logic and effectiveness but whose proper functioning is necessarily destructive of human health. Indeed, if such expressions were used, they would probably tend to be heard as meaning a war with few or no injuries, an epidemic with no deaths, and so on. Thus, from these cases it would seem that, with respect to nonliving things, the judgment of health will have its literal meaning as an evaluation of the effects on or conditions of positive individual health if it possibly can, as in the case of a

society, an economy, a town, and so forth. When it cannot
have its literal meaning, it will be clearly understood as an
ironic and, in these cases only, a metaphorical usage.

Fourth, and finally, the claim that such a phrase as "a
healthy city" is a metaphor leads us directly into a distressing
dilemma, for it requires that something that contains or includes people can be metaphorically healthy only if it systemically makes many of the people in it literally unhealthy.
In other words, in such cases the analogy that can be abstracted from the concept health must necessarily contradict
the literal meaning of health. But this is certainly absurd,
just as it would be to say that a bank can be friendly only if
many of the people in it are unfriendly.

The real issue here is that when a judgment of health is
made, even in the sense of proper functioning, it necessarily
includes an evaluation of the working order of all of the parts
of the functioning whole. Thus, in the case of a city or a
business—something whose proper functioning includes the
structured and systematic activity of human beings—such a
judgment must include an evaluation of proper *organic* functioning, even *human* functioning, which is, of course, the
literal use of the notion of health. That is, the idea of a
healthy city can only make sense as an extension of the
literal, nonmetaphorical use of health. In the case of a car or
a television set, on the other hand, no such literal meaning is
involved in an attribution of health, so that the notion of
proper functioning is simply abstracted away and applied
metaphorically. With respect to the judgments we are discussing—the judgments of our own cities, businesses, economy, and the like—there is the further problem that an extension of the literal meaning of health seems clearly to
entail the systematic denial of health to many or most of the
human beings who are participating in those groups and
organizations. Thus, if this usage of health is not a metaphor,

then either the judgment is simply mistaken or the normal meaning of health must in some sense be self-contradictory.

This brings us to the central problem, but first we must clarify exactly what kind of judgment health is if it is neither metaphorical nor strictly literal. I believe it must be a literal judgment, but not in the absolute sense of the garden, where a healthy society, garden, or preserve means healthy people, plants, and animals. Rather it is literal in the relative sense that the people in the society, economy, or city are about as healthy as could be expected. To judge these institutions as healthy is to say that they are providing a more or less maximally healthy context for individual life, that this is all that can be expected from institutions, and that all other health matters are essentially up to the individual, the doctors, chance, and so forth. Used in this way, the judgment of health is applied to institutions in the same way that it is applied to attitudes and diets: it rests on a final judgment of its contribution to the health of the individual beings involved. But because it is a judgment about organizations that include humans, as opposed to plants or animals, it can have a unique meaning. The ordinary judgment about the health of plants or animals is generally a straightforward physical and biological one. But, as we have seen, the ordinary judgment of human health is more complex, necessarily including, as it does, a reference to both the physiological and the moral aspects of human life, the realm of physical health and the realm of mental health. Since it is quintessentially human both to make and to be held responsible for choices, an individual's ability to make responsible choices must be part of an evaluation of his or her health. And one of the obvious things that individuals can *to some degree* make choices about and be held responsible for is their own health.

Thus, in the judgment of an institution it is not immediately clear to what degree the institution and not the individual has responsibility—that is, to what degree it can be meaningfully judged with respect to the health of its members—whereas in a garden or a preserve the individual plant or animal cannot be held responsible for its own health in the same way, so that the judgment of the organization is much more straightforward. Since humans are both physiological units and moral actors, an evaluation of both components must be included in any judgment of health, whether of individuals or of systems of individuals. But with respect to systems or institutions, a prior decision must be made, a standard set, in order to establish the grounds on which the judgment will be made, to establish to what degree the system or institution is subject to judgment—is liable—for the health of the individuals. On this interpretation, then, the health of a society, an economy depends upon the degree to which it maximizes its contribution to the health of its members within the limits of its impact on the health of those individuals, limits set by a prior analysis of the respective responsibilities.

A healthy society is one that maximizes as far as possible the health of its members, and, as we have seen, a healthy individual is one who can achieve personal control through a combination of moral responsibility and physiological functioning. Thus, a healthy society allows maximum personal control—that is, moral and physical effectiveness—for its members. In the judgments we have seen, this is what is being claimed about our economy, about Houston, and so on. And because this claim is made seriously, with full knowledge that these same institutions are directly causing widespread physical and mental illness (as well as even greater loss of effective control through the degradation of work and welfare and the bureaucratic mindlessness of modern life), it implies the judgment that these conditions of poor health are inevitable, that, all things considered, the individuals involved are about as healthy as is possible, since the institutions have maximized the conditions for individual health. In other words, the claim that the institutions are healthy is the same as the claim that the poor health that does exist is essentially the responsibility of the individuals who suffer it, a claim that is obviously compatible with and supportive of the practice of modern medicine. Furthermore, to claim, as the doctors and theorists do, that poor health in our society is a matter only of individual bodies and self-directed actions is to claim that our institutions are healthy and have no further responsibility. The social and political implications of the concept of health are contained in the very claim that it has no such implications.

This claim, then, rests on a prior assumption about the limits of institutional impact on health: that maximizing the conditions for human health entails systemic institutional responsibility for immense human suffering. Put another way, this means that for the institutions to promote general health, they must also promote a great deal of unhealth, and this obviously means that either the judgment is simply wrong or there is a contradiction somewhere in the idea of health itself. Since the makers of these judgments do not think they are wrong, they are necessarily pointing to a contradiction, which must exist somewhere between the two components of human health: moral responsibility and physiological functioning. Since the evidence for excessive and unnecessary physical illness is apparent, the idea seems to be (and is, as we shall see) that in order for the institutions to promote moral health, to maximize the possibilities for everyone to have a fully human life, they must also promote activities and organizations that will be harmful to the physical health, even the moral health, of a significant number of individuals, usually a specific group or groups of individuals. In other words, in order to provide the opportunity for general hu-

man health, particularly general moral health, many severe
sacrifices of both mental and physical health will have to be
made by a large part of the population. The assumption is
made that social health requires systemic and systematic individual suffering, that it is incompatible with whatever conditions would be required for inclusive individual health.
This is what is meant when *Newsweek*, after mentioning the
crime, the pollution, the poverty, and the racism, ends its
article on Houston with the comment:

> None of these problems looms very large to Houston's
> bustling middle class. If prosperity has its price, in the
> city of the fast buck most people are only too willing to
> pay it.

Thus, the middle class and, presumably, the upper class
enjoy Houston's health, while everyone, and particularly the
lower classes, suffer the somehow necessary consequences
for individual health.

CHAPTER SEVEN

SOCIAL THEORY AND HEALTH
The Assumed Contradiction

Thus far, I have suggested that most judgments of social or institutional health are problematic because, owing to a prior analysis of social life and social institutions, they assume there is a contradiction, either at the individual level or at the social level, between the requirements for the moral and the physiological health of individual human beings. For this analysis of inherent contradiction to be correct, the concept of health itself would have to be internally contradictory: we would have to be able to say reasonably and meaningfully that by one action we can both promote health and destroy health, and this is simply not the case. We may use the term in contradictory ways, but that is because we are confused about its meaning in certain situations, due to the historically dominant ideology of medical science, or because we simply make an incorrect judgment owing to lack of full information, bias, or whatever. But the fundamental criteria by which we judge human health are not logically contradictory; indeed, they are quite consistent, readily apparent, and used meaningfully in everyday communication. The seeming contradiction between the doctors' idea of health and our everyday understanding of it only means that the doctors have, for historical and political reasons, made a mistake, not that the concept is incoherent.

Nevertheless, most modern social, economic, and psychological theories share the general assumption, though it is

expressed in different ways, that the proper or necessary—
the healthy—functioning of a society and its institutions requires the systematic denial of the essential human needs,
the health, of many if not all of its members. A good example is a sentence from a newspaper article on terrorism
by a political science professor: "Any healthy society contains
a number of students who are disquieted by the injustices of
that society . . ." (Richard Clutterbuck, *Los Angeles Times*,
Dec. 1, 1977). Here it is assumed that a healthy society
contains injustices; either they are inevitable in it or they are
necessary for it. But this author clearly means systematic
injustices (he refers to Vietnam, racism, economic exploitation, women's oppression), and since injustice means the
selective denial of human needs, the arbitrary denial of effective personal control, it follows that in this view a healthy
society is one that makes some of its citizens systematically
unhealthy.

The necessity of this conflict between a society and its
members has been generally accepted in Western social
thought since at least the Renaissance. Isaiah Berlin finds it
to have been first announced by Machiavelli, though both
Plato and Aristotle felt that the proper working of a society
required the oppression of some of its members. The scientific conception of natural, immutable, and necessary laws
that regulate all of nature was translated into social theory
first by Hobbes and later by the social scientists, with the
result that the necessity of individual suffering was legitimated through the idea that human society and its institutions
operate according to their own necessary and objective laws,
laws that work independently of and even in conflict with the
needs of individual human beings. This notion of objective
laws that can be known scientifically provided a dual certainty
at the basis of all subsequent social analysis: the scientific
commitment to the existence of such morally neutral laws,

and the more universal and fundamental certainty, instinctively felt but not well articulated, of the basic moral and physical needs of individual human life, the requirements of human health. Inevitably, these two certainties were found to be in conflict—inevitable because, first of all, by definition objective laws are external to and coercive of individual actions and, second, because these laws were sought to explain and legitimate a new social order, one whose institutions were soon recognized as excessively debilitating to the health of many thousands of people. This dualism at the basis of "scientific" social thought has resulted in the general conviction that a viable society must induce suffering among some of its people, usually among a particular economic class. Social health contradicts individual health to some degree, and thus it is here that the apparent conflicts in our judgments of health arise.

At the very beginning of modern social thought, Hobbes formulated the conflict clearly: "law and right differ as much as obligation and liberty; which in one and the same matter are inconsistent" (Hobbes, p. 109). In general, Hobbes, Locke, and Rousseau assumed this conflict when they conceptualized the social contract as something that separates the free and rational individual from the restrictive but necessary society. It permeates John Stuart Mill's defense of individual liberty as against the oppression of society: "there needs protection . . . against the tendency of society . . . to fetter the development, and, if possible, prevent the formation, of any individuality not in harmony with its ways, and compels all characters to fashion themselves upon the model of its own" (Mill and Bentham, p. 479).

But it is in the writings of the social and psychological theorists who laid the foundations of modern social science that the truly oppressive nature of society and its laws is most fully and "objectively" developed. For Durkheim, probably the most academically influential of the great social theorists, society is an external entity that coerces and constrains individuals for its own needs and for their own good:

> Now society also gives us the sensation of a perpetual dependence. Since it has a nature which is peculiar to itself and different from our individual nature, it pursues ends which are likewise special to it; but, as it cannot attain them except through our intermediacy, it imperiously demands our aid. It requires that, forgetful of our own interest, we make ourselves its servitors, and it submits us to every sort of inconvenience, privation and sacrifice, without which social life would be impossible. It is because of this that at every instant we are obliged to submit ourselves to rules of conduct which are sometimes even contrary to our most fundamental inclinations and instincts. (Durkheim, 1965, p. 237)

However, as Durkheim points out, the privation and sacrifice are generally borne by the lower class, a class formed by the division of labor and determined in a "normal" or "healthy" society on the basis of inferior natural abilities. "[L]abor is divided spontaneously only if society is constituted in such a way that social inequalities exactly express natural inequalities" (Durkheim, 1964, p. 377). These "natural inequalities" are based on the difference between the "useful and deserving" and the "mediocre and incapable" (Durkheim, 1951, p. 261). A "normal" society enforces the class privation of the inferior people through the force of moral coercion, and the deprived individuals, with some sick exceptions, will be content.

> It will be said that it is not always sufficient to make men content, that there are some men whose desires go

> beyond their faculties. This is true, but these are ex-
> ceptional and, one may say, morbid cases. (Durkheim,
> 1964, p. 376)

Thus, social oppression is necessary and must be borne by
the individuals of the lower class, who will be morally co-
erced into believing that the institutional commitment to
their own social inferiority is natural. For Durkheim the
necessity and acceptance of this systematic effort to convince
one group that it should be denied the life possibilities available to others constitutes the basic social function of the
division of labor and thus determines the health of the society:

> The division of labor does not present individuals to
> one another, but social functions. And society is inter-
> ested in the play of the latter; in so far as they regu-
> larly concur, or do not concur, it will be healthy or ill.
> (Durkheim, 1964, p. 407)

This assumption of the conflict between institutions and
individuals, and of the inevitable class-located manifestation
of this conflict, is perhaps most categorical in Durkheim, but
it is also clear in the social theories of Max Weber. Weber's
understanding of social life is more historical, and he is more
concerned with human actions than human individuals, but
the sense of an inherent conflict between human needs and
industrial social life underlies his analysis. It is expressed in
his deep personal pessimism as well as in his description of
the increasing routinization of social life, and it is fundamental to what is perhaps his central concept: the idea of
"rational action." For Weber rational action is opposed to irrational, affective, and traditional actions in that it is conscious, controlled, and productive, that is, constitutively human. Further, the concept also indicates action that has its

own logic and momentum and that has come to operate
more and more independently of human needs. The ambiguity of the concept (and the consequent image of inherent
conflict) is apparent in his discussion of bureaucracy, where
he connects the objective efficiency of bureaucracy with the
intense rationality of the market economy and the capitalist
enterprise and shows that they are fundamentally opposed to
many basic human needs:

> Bureaucratization offers above all the optimum possi-
> bility for carrying through the principle of specializing
> administrative functions according to purely objective
> considerations. . . . The "objective" discharge of busi-
> ness primarily means a discharge of business according
> to *calculable rules* and "without regard for persons."
> "Without regard for persons" is also the watchword of
> the "market" and, in general, of all pursuits of naked
> economic interests. . . . Normally, the very large, mod-
> ern capitalist enterprises are themselves unequalled
> models of strict bureaucratic organization. . . . Its spe-
> cific nature, which is welcomed by capitalism, develops
> the more perfectly the more the bureaucracy is "de-
> humanized," the more completely it succeeds in elim-
> inating from official business love, hatred, and all
> purely personal, irrational, and emotional elements
> which escape calculation. This is the specific nature
> of bureaucracy and is appraised as its special virtue.
> (Weber, pp. 215–216)

According to Weber, this deep conflict of economic rationality with human life, with human rationality and human
health, has become an essential condition of modern social
life:

> Where the bureaucratization of administration has been
> completely carried through, a form of power relation is
> established that is practically unshatterable. . . . More

and more the material fate of the masses depends upon
the steady and correct functioning of the increasingly
bureaucratic organizations of private capitalism. The
idea of eliminating these organizations becomes more
and more utopian. (p. 229)

Thus, as with Durkheim, a conflict that is socially apparent is
analyzed as being socially inevitable, and the "correct functioning" of social institutions both determines the "material
fate" and requires the dehumanization of groups of people.

Through the work of Freud this conflict has been built not
only into our modern understanding of social institutions but
also into our understanding of human psychology. In analyzing the determinants and conditions of psychic health, Freud
decided that there is an absolute and inherent contradiction
between the needs of individuals and the needs of society,
and he stated it forcefully:

Our civilization is largely responsible for our misery. . . .
(Freud, 1961, p. 33)

A person becomes neurotic because he cannot tolerate
the amount of frustration which society imposes on him
in the service of its cultural ideals. . . . (p. 34)

The price we pay for our advance in civilization is a loss
of happiness through the heightening of the sense of
guilt. (p. 81)

So . . . the two urges, the one towards personal happiness and the other towards union with other human
beings must struggle with each other in every individual; and so, also, the two processes of individual and of
cultural development must stand in hostile opposition
to each other and mutually dispute the ground. (p. 88)

Underlying all these visions of inevitable conflict and necessary suffering is the more fundamental idea that the re-

quirements for the moral health of individuals are essentially incompatible with the requirements for the proper functioning of a society. Though these theorists and their followers have many different views on the bases of human motivation, all of them more or less recognize that human beings are characterized by their ability and their need both to make conscious choices—conscious in the sense that they are based on a coherent and reliable understanding of an ongoing social and natural world—and to take effective actions —effective in the sense that chosen actions will be more or less successful in the achievement of personal and social goals. The possibility of such choices and actions creates the concrete experience of moral responsibility and personal control, that is, the experience of moral health. But these theorists uniformly build into their analyses of institutions the assumption that our modern society cannot satisfy, for *all* its members at least, the needs for both conscious choices and effective actions, because at bottom these seem to be conceptually separate demands and cannot mutually coexist; like the poles of a magnet, when one is present, the other must be absent.

In order to understand the basis for this assumption, we must examine these concepts further. The way these theorists use them, or, rather, fail to use them, hides the drama of the individual's confrontation with society. First of all, for choices to be truly *conscious,* the coherent and reliable understanding on which they are based must in turn be based on a coherent and reliable social order (the natural order is not considered to be a problem in this regard). In such a social context each individual will know with relative confidence the relevant aspects, the available options, and the likely consequences of his or her actions. The stable social order, that is, more or less guarantees the present and future contexts of choices, so that our conscious efforts to consider all possibilities will be generally successful. Without such a guarantee, in a more problematic and capricious social context, our choices will necessarily become more arbitrary and desperate and therefore less conscious. Real human choice, then, requires a well-ordered society, and such a society requires a strong sense of moral coherence and shared social commitments. The people of the society must actively and naturally support its procedures and institutions, for without this support the social order must be imposed, and conflict and uncertainty will result.

On the other hand, the ability to take *effective* actions means that an individual can act on the world successfully so as to satisfy the basic needs of human life as they are expressed in his or her particular social and cultural goals. This ability characterizes the practical, or physical, aspects of human life. As individuals we must be able to satisfy such direct needs as food and sex and communication, and we must be able to arrange the material world so that these needs, as well as the need to feel confident of their continued satisfaction, are met. We conceptualize the world, we analyze possibilities and make conscious choices, as members of a social group; but we act on the world, we physically and mentally survive in the world, as individuals. Together, then, these two aspects of human life constitute the characteristically human need for the experience of *essential* personal control. Without either a coherent social context or the possibility of effective material actions, a person cannot control the satisfaction of his or her human needs, and thus that person cannot be healthy.

It is here, then, that the inherent polarity of human life is found, according to the main tradition of social science, and the critical issue is: What are the *essential* needs of individuals? It is assumed that for any human being the "natural" satisfaction of these essential needs entails the systematic denial of those same needs to others. As individuals our deepest and most definitive impulses are seen to be in support of our efforts to manipulate and oppress others in order to guarantee the effectiveness of our own physical actions, the accomplishment of our "essential" goals. Thus our own humanity as individuals necessitates a fundamental effort toward social inhumanity. Moreover, if all of us follow these impulses, we will even oppress ourselves: oppression will be widespread, the social order will be disrupted, and clear conscious choices will no longer be possible. In other words, our natural human efforts as individuals to achieve effective action inevitably contradict our equally natural and human need to live in a coherent and reliable society, to make conscious choices. And although our efforts to share a social commitment and a moral understanding are as intense and deepseated as our efforts to achieve effective action, fulfillment of the former would necessitate a severe restriction on our ability to act effectively as individuals to satisfy our essential desires. Thus, at the very basis of what it means to be human, we contradict ourselves. Our own most fundamental efforts to achieve meaningful personal control over our own lives require the denial of effective personal control to others and thus, inevitably, the denial of conscious control to ourselves.

The formulations of this essential human conflict vary. Durkheim saw society as something external to and coercive of individuals and therefore found the conflict to be between the natural but destructive desires of individuals and the humanizing constraints of a social order and its moral system, virtually any social order and virtually any moral system.

> But how determine the quantity of well-being, comfort
> or luxury legitimately to be craved by a human being?
> Nothing appears in man's organic nor in his psychologi-

cal constitution which sets a limit to such tendencies.
. . . It is not human nature which can assign the vari-
able limits necessary to our needs. They are thus unlimited so far as they depend on the individual alone.
Irrespective of any external regulatory force, our capacity for feeling is in itself an insatiable and bottomless
abyss. . . .
. . . But if nothing external can restrain this capacity,
it can only be a source of torment to itself. Unlimited
desires are insatiable by definition and insatiability
is rightly considered a sign of morbidity. (Durkheim,
1951, p. 247)

Here we can see the assumption of inherent conflict, even of
inherent unhealth. Society can control the conflict and provide health, but only by severely constraining the natural
desires of the individual. Conscious choices, that is, must
strongly oppose the basic impulses toward effective actions.

For Freud the conflict is not between the individual and
society but within the psyche of the individual. All of us seek
pleasure instinctively, and that pleasure can be achieved,
weakly, through the sublimation of sex into love, art, morality, and the building of civilization, or it can be achieved,
strongly, through the mistreatment and destruction of other
people, even of ourselves. "[A] satisfaction of instinct spells
happiness for us . . ." (Freud, 1961, p. 25), and the most
powerful of those instincts leads an individual to view his or
her neighbor as: "someone who tempts them to satisfy their
aggressiveness on him, to exploit his capacity for work without compensation, to use him sexually without his consent,
to seize his possessions, to humiliate him, to cause him pain,
to torture and to kill him" (Freud, 1961, p. 58). We are
caught in the battle of Eros (conscious choice, social stability)
and Thanatos (effective individual action), and thus we must
expect a great deal of pain and suffering.

Weber also finds an inherent conflict at the basis of human

life, but his analysis is more subtle and his description somewhat less melodramatic. For him all individual human actions can be divided into two more or less exclusive and
exhaustive types: communal action and societal action. As he
defines and uses them, these types of action characterize
only the abstract and polarized possibilities of any individual
action, so that they cut across his historical categories and
thus provide the basis for a general analysis of social life.

> Communal action refers to that action which is oriented
> to the feeling of the actors that they belong together.
> Societal action, on the other hand, is oriented to a ra-
> tionally motivated adjustment of interest. (Weber,
> p. 183)

Communal action is based on considerations of "social hon-
or." That is, it is oriented toward moral coherence and social
participation, and since "*status groups* are normally com-
munities" (p. 256), it is the type of action that characterizes a
sense of "status." Societal action, on the other hand, is the
type of rationally self-interested action that corresponds to
the rational and calculable workings of the market, and since
"'class situation' is . . . ultimately 'market situation'" (p.
252), this type of action underlies the recognition of "class"
location, that is, the recognition of the need for effective
individual action, through the market, in order to satisfy
economic, that is, material, interests. Through these concepts, Weber opposes the satisfaction of individual needs to
the satisfaction of social commitments, since "the rationally
motivated adjustment of interest" always conflicts with "the
feeling of actors that they belong together."

> In contrast to the purely economically determined "class
> situation" we wish to designate as "status situation"
> every typical component of the life fate of men that is

determined by a specific, positive or negative, social
estimation of *honor*. . . . (pp. 186–187)

Now "status groups" hinder the strict carrying through
of the sheer market principle. . . . (p. 185)

The principle of status stratification is in opposition
to a distribution of power which is regulated exclusively
through the market. (p. 192)

As we have seen, once societal action has been institutionalized into capitalism and bureaucracy, its natural effects of
leveling status honor and dehumanizing society become, for
all practical purposes, irreversible. Under the heading, "The
permanent character of the bureaucratic machine," Weber
writes: "Under otherwise equal conditions, a 'societal action,'
which is methodically ordered and led, is superior to every
resistance of 'mass' or even of 'communal action'" (p. 228).
Thus, the conflict of people with their society is inevitable,
at least in the modern world, and for Weber, as for Freud, it
stems from a polarization at the source of human action.
Material individual needs oppose social identity, but in
Weber this takes an interesting turn. In his analysis it is
effective action for the satisfaction of individual needs, the
rational adjustment of interests, that leads to a rational society and efficient institutions, while it is the desire for moral
and social involvement that seeks to limit rigorous social
coherence in favor of a more personal and human, even
more arbitrary, social life. Effective action leads, through
increasing rationality, to absolute social coherence, but this
coherence, through its own rationality, denies the possibility
of effective individual actions, at least for most of us. The
polarity is reversed: rather than the overriding strength of
our individual desires constantly threatening to disrupt our
ever tenuous moral and social coherence, the certainty of
our conscious understanding is decisive and crushes our in-

dividuality. In this sense Weber is closer to Mill and Adam Smith than to Durkheim and Freud. But the mutually exclusive poles are still there. Whatever the variations in analysis, throughout this tradition of social theory the essential requirements of human life, the needs for social participation and for individuality, are seen to be inherently contradictory.

More recently this tradition has been continued through such social scientific statements as these by Gerhard Lenski:

> In most instances, the interests of the individual will be subversive of the interests of the society, and vice versa. . . . Logically, it is not possible for the interests of society to be compatible with the interests of all of its members. . . . Under such conditions, the most that is possible is that the interests of society are consistent with the interests of *some* of its members. (Lenski, p. 35)

> Human societies are such imperfect systems. Their members frequently work at cross-purposes with one another, and the actions of the whole are often harmful to the parts. . . . We are obliged to define as the goals of a given society *those ends toward which the more or less coordinated efforts of the whole are directed— without regard to the harm they may do to many individual members, even the majority.* (p. 41, his italics)

Here the assumption of inherent contradiction, even the explicit implication that good social health necessitates bad individual health among some social groups, is clear. In other cases the essentially moral assumptions about the nature of social life are more carefully hidden behind obscure terminology and an appearance of overwhelming scholarly detachment. Talcott Parsons, for example, offers his famous pattern variables as logical dichotomies that represent the universal and fundamental dilemmas of social life that all individuals must confront. Each of us, that is, can orient ourselves and our actions toward one side or the other of the dichotomy but not to both. One of these five inherent and necessary dichotomies is the putatively logical distinction—and thus inevitable conflict—between a "self-orientation" and a "collectivity-orientation." According to Parsons, in other words, it is a given of social life that we cannot orient our actions toward our individual needs and toward the needs of our society at the same time.

Seymour Martin Lipset, among others, has used this conception of pattern variables, and the self-collectivity conflict in particular, to argue that social stability, together with democracy, civil liberties, and tolerance for political deviance —that is, a "healthy" society—are best achieved in a society in which an elite class governs and essentially controls the rest of the population, who "cannot be expected to understand" the rules by which they are governed.

> Perhaps the highest degree of tolerance for political deviance is found, therefore, in democratic systems which are most strongly characterized by the values of elitism and diffuseness. . . . It is deferential respect for the elite . . . which underlies the vaunted freedom of dissent in countries like Britain and Sweden . . . civil liberties will be stronger in elitist democracies. . . . Thus, the values of elitism and ascription may protect an operating democracy from the excesses of populism and may facilitate the acceptance by the privileged strata of the welfare planning state, whereas emphases on self-orientation and anti-elitism may be conducive to right-wing populism. (Lipset, p. 170)

But Lipset recognizes that the lower strata will suffer because of this elitism:

> Elitism in the status hierarchy has major dysfunctions
> which should be noted here. . . . A system of differen-
> tial status rankings requires that a large proportion of
> the population accept a negative conception of their
> own worth as compared with others in more privileged
> positions. To be socially defined as being low according
> to a system of values, which one respects, must mean
> that, to some unspecified degree, such low status is
> experienced as "punishment" in a psychological sense.
> This felt sense of deprivation or punishment is often
> manifested in "self-hatred." . . . (p. 170)

He might also mention, of course, that low status tends to
make people physically ill as well. Since social stability and
elitism are fundamental values of a good society, and since
excessive individual suffering might cause instability, it is
necessary somehow to adjust the lower classes to their own
deprivation and suffering so that they will not disrupt the
"healthy" social order.

> There are different adaptive mechanisms which have
> emerged to reconcile low status individuals to their po-
> sitions and thus contribute to the stability and legiti-
> macy of the larger system. The three most common ap-
> pear to be:
>   1. *Religion:* Belief in a religion . . . which emphasizes
> the possibility or even the probability that the poor on
> earth will enjoy higher status in heaven or in a reincar-
> nation, operates to adjust them to their station, and
> motivates those in low positions to carry out their role
> requirements.
>   2. *Social mobility:* The belief that achievement is pos-
> sible . . . provides stabilizing functions comparable to
> those suggested for religion.
>   3. *Political action:* . . . also helps to adjust the de-
> prived groups to their situation. (p. 170)

Thus, although the suffering of large groups of the society is necessary, these people can, through myths and promises, be reconciled into accepting their suffering as reasonable.

All of these theorists derive the inevitable contradiction between social health and general individual health from the assumption that individual human beings are essentially autonomous, self-seeking creatures whose individual interests are by nature opposed to the interests of society. Lenski, Parsons, and Lipset, following Durkheim, emphasize the idea of overall social interests—the requirements of social stability, the possibility of conscious choices—as the necessary barrier to the satisfaction of the needs and desires of at least some groups of individuals. Other theorists follow Hobbes and Freud in deemphasizing the role of "society" as such and concentrating on the inherent antagonism and hostility of individuals toward one another. The sociologist Milton Gordon, for example, offers an analysis of human nature in which he postulates that:

> . . . the forces making for aggression and hostile feelings and thus laying the groundwork for aggressive behavior lie pervasively in the human environment and in ourselves. Thus we are faced with that complex mixture of cooperation and aggressive feeling and behavior which makes up the tension-laden human scene. It is this tension, provided by the interaction of every man's "human nature" with every other man's "human nature" that constitutes the most telling aspect of society and social institutions. (Gordon, p. 63)

Sociologist Randall Collins, believes that

> human beings are sociable but conflict-prone animals. . . . Each individual is basically pursuing his own interests and . . . there are many situations, notably ones

where power is involved, in which those interests are
inherently antagonistic. (Collins, pp. 59–60)

And social psychologist Elliot Aronson tells us more simply
and directly: Man is an aggressive animal. . . . I would
define aggression as a behavior aimed at causing harm or
pain (Aronson, pp. 142–143).

This concern with aggression and with human beings as
animals reflects the recent influence of ethology, the study
of animal behavior, on social theory. After careful observations of how different species of animals organize, reproduce, nourish themselves, and interact among themselves
and with other animals, the ethologists have claimed that
these different types of activities can be understood as manifestations of universal animal instincts, which in some sense
"cause" or "direct" the specific behavior of each individual
animal. Some go on to claim that since human beings are
also "animals," much or most of our individual behavior must
also be understood as instinctual in nature. "These deepest
strata of the human personality are, in their dynamics, not
essentially different from the instincts of animals . . ." (Lorenz, p. 248). This conception of our underlying animal instincts can play the same role in generating social theory as
has the Freudian conception of our basic sexual instincts or
even as have the assumptions about our "natural" desires
and motivations by such theorists as Hobbes, Rousseau, and
Rawls. Thus, claims about our fundamental "animal nature"
are coming more and more to replace the earlier claims
about our fundamental "human nature," perhaps because the
evidence about animal instincts seems somewhat more empirical and objective than the more traditional claims about
human instincts and interests.

Yet the understanding of these animal instincts and the

image of the specific types of social action they determine or instruct are not noticeably different from the idea of human instincts and drives—intense self-interest, innate aggression, and a marginally controllable and thus constantly threatening degree of individual hostility toward other individuals and groups—that Freud, Hobbes, and others assumed as fundamental to individual behavior. As Lorenz puts it, "the destructive intensity of the aggression drive, still a hereditary evil of mankind . . . springs 'spontaneously' from the inner human being . . ." (Lorenz, pp. 42, 50). According to Ardrey:

> Aggressiveness, natural to all living beings, is the determined pursuit of one's interests. And aggressiveness becomes violent only with physical threat and assault. . . . Yet the propensity for violence . . . exists like a layer of buried molten magma underlying all human topography, seeking unceasingly some unimportant fissure to become the most magnificent of volcanoes. (Ardrey, pp. 284, 279)

The ethologists go on to argue that aggression is beneficial to all animals, including humans, because it maximizes their ability to survive, both as individuals and as a species. Aggression in all other animals does not lead to social disorder and rampant destructiveness, but among humans, because we have language and culture as well as instincts, it is somehow more likely to overrun its instinctual limits.

> All the great dangers threatening humanity with extinction are direct consequences of conceptual thought and verbal speech. They drove man out of the paradise in which he could follow his instincts with impunity. . . . (Lorenz, p. 238)

Once again, a conflict between the instinctual needs of individuals and the conditions for a stable social life is portrayed as inevitable. Ardrey even argues that enjoyment of violence is a normal human response and not the result of individual neurosis. He concludes: "Were we truly sick societies, then I suggest that the violent way might be more easily containable; it is because we are healthy that we are in trouble" (Ardrey, p. 286).

The ethologists study animal behavior and derive general conclusions about human instincts and the corresponding contradictions of social life. The social theorists adopt and adapt these conclusions as basic assumptions from which to begin an analysis of the logic and direction of social interaction and institutions. Thus, the acceptance of an inherent contradiction between individual needs and social stability, between individual health and social health, is built solidly into the work of these social theorists. And for these theorists the "scientific" study of animal behavior has provided a seemingly legitimate foundation on which to rest that assumption. As it turns out, however, the claims of the ethologists, like other images about "human nature," cannot withstand much scrutiny. In the first place, the evidence itself is unclear. Ethologists and zoologists who are not inclined to generalize so quickly from animal life to human life have raised severe objections. Without entering into debates about data and their interpretation, it can be pointed out that a theoretical leap from animal behavior to human actions is logically untenable. As Lorenz and others have recognized, the ability of humans to use language, to think conceptually, interferes decisively with the direct manifestations of animal instincts, whatever they may be. At this point the argument contradicts itself, for on what basis can the claim be made that language and culture can override the instincts that protect us from aggression but not the instincts of aggression themselves? It seems apparent that we can *choose* our actions—that is, we can choose to be aggressive or not—in a way that animals cannot. The biological similarity and the implications of evolution are interesting, but they are important to an understanding of ourselves and our society only to the extent that we begin to understand their relation to the possibility of language, culture, and conscious choice, something the ethologists are manifestly not trying to do. Rather, they simply notice that both animals and humans act aggressively and proceed to claim that all these acts are essentially the same and that they arise from the same origin. Having made this obviously simplifying assumption, the social theorists can proceed apace, firm in their conviction that the basic sources and goals of human behavior have been universally identified. But this conviction entails a strong theoretical commitment to the relative unimportance of language and conceptual thought as basic factors in the generation and thus the understanding of human social life. Collins, for example, states such a position explicitly:

> Man is an animal; "human society" means a group of animals meeting each other, communicating through basic animal gestures for sex, parenthood, threat, submission, mutual support, and play. Our human capacity for symbolism only adds refinements to the basic gestures, however powerful they may be in their consequences for the number of persons who can live together and the complexity of the things they can do. (Collins, p. 92)

> the talking animal has social ties below the level of verbal meaning, and his motives largely reside there as well. (p. 111)

Neither Collins nor the ethologists can explain how language can both make us distinctively human and be so deci-

sively unimportant for an understanding of our human lives
and actions. Their argument must finally reduce to the claim
that, since individual actions are decisively instinctual, conceptual thought can enable us to understand the sources of
those actions but cannot enable us to affect, change, and
control those actions significantly, an argument that may be
true with respect to our understanding of the behavior of
animals but one that is not obviously true, and even apparently false, with respect to understanding our own actions. Both the ethologists and the ethological social theorists can only assume (since they do not address the issue)
an answer to the complex and difficult question of the relation between consciousness and biology, between conceptual
thought and physical movements, the mind and the body.
Their simple assumption is that the body is decisively dominant with respect to basic social actions, and then they add
the essentially moral assumption that our crucial instinctual
needs require us to be aggressive, socially disruptive, and
harmful to others. Because we are animals who have somehow learned to think and talk, it seems that we are necessarily contradictory to ourselves. And once again social
health is "instinctually" incompatible with general individual
health.

Some theorists from the emerging discipline of sociobiology have presented a new and much more biologically sophisticated version of the ethological argument. According to
them, genes, not instincts, make both animals and humans
aggressive, hostile, and selfish. Sociobiology is a version of
evolutionary theory that puts every individual animal—and
for some theorists, humans—under the behavioral direction
of the programming of that individual's genes to reproduce
themselves and thus to reproduce and evolve the species.
Since each set of genes is inevitably competing with all other
sets of genes in this eternal struggle to reproduce themselves

and then to survive and reproduce again, every complete gene machine—that is, every individual animal—is genetically locked into competitive, aggressive, and self-interested behavior. Naturally society, particularly human society, will be nasty and brutish, at least to the extent that the genes have their way. As Richard Dawkins admonishes in *The Selfish Gene*:

> My own feeling is that a human society based simply on the gene's law of universal ruthless selfishness would be a very nasty society in which to live. But unfortunately, however much we may deplore something, it does not stop it being true. . . . Be warned that if you wish, as I do, to build a society in which individuals cooperate generously and unselfishly towards a common good, you can expect little help from biological nature. Let us try to *teach* generosity and altruism, because we are born selfish. (Dawkins, p. 3)

Other sociobiologists, including David Barash and even Dawkins later in his book, point out that although this evolutionary idea of the gene provides a good basis for the analysis of animal behavior, it is not clearly applicable to the analysis of human societies. There is simply no reason to assume that as human beings our ability for conceptual thought and conscious control is fundamentally subject to our biology, whether in terms of instincts or genes. The assumption that it is, whether in sociobiology or ethology, must remain essentially arbitrary and prescriptive because it is derived from a commitment to certain social values rather than from any demonstrable evidence about human life.

All of these social theories—from Hobbes to sociobiology —are built upon an image of a basic human nature that underlies all individual actions. Such an image consists of claims about the essential interests, drives, desires, and needs that universally and necessarily motivate all human beings. Some such idea, is necessary for any social theory, for without it we would never be able to understand, in the sense of making a good ballpark prediction, what any particular individual might do when faced with a new and unexpected situation. In other words, if human action is theoretically understandable, as we are assuming it to be, it must be based on some general and abstract principles, some universal motivations that inform all individual activity. In any specific social theory these motivations must not only be implicitly or explicitly assumed to be present, they must also be given a definite behavioral content as a basis for the conceptions and predictions of the theory. Such content has, as we have seen, ranged from competitive self-interest and innate but rational hostility through insatiable desire for gratification to sexual lust and instinctual aggression. It has also occasionally been seen as innate kindness, altruism, and sociability, as in the works of Rousseau, Marx, and, to some degree, Weber. Whatever it is found to be by a particular theorist, it alerts both us and the theory to what human beings *really* are, what they *really* want, stripped of all their historical and cultural trappings. From this information we can construct an idea of what social institutions and social interaction must be like, of how social life can be developed and must be limited in certain ways according to the nature of things. Indeed, such a construction is logically contained within any particular conception of human nature itself, for knowing what the fundamental motivations and needs of human beings are is the same thing as knowing what kind of social life they are capable of creating. Thus, the image of human nature contains the social theory in germ, and, accordingly, that image is a moral one, for it prescribes how individuals can and will treat one another naturally; therefore, it inevitably suggests, implicitly or explicitly, what a society should accept as normal behavior and what it should prohibit and control as abnormal behavior.

The notion of human nature, then, is offered as a fact about human beings, but it implies a moral conclusion, a statement defining what social values are compatible with the facts of human life. The next question, of course, is where do those facts come from, and, as I have tried to show, they inevitably come from moral assumptions disguised as empirical certainty. The phrase "human nature" seems to indicate a connection between human life and the nature of things, that is, natural science. As such, it works as a tacit theoretical attitude that serves to legitimate psychological and behavioral assumptions about human motivations, that is, moral assumptions, as natural facts. Of course, there are clear facts about human beings, specifically, the facts that connect them with all other animals—the facts of their biological processes—and the fact that distinguishes them from all other animals—the fact that they use a language and communicate conceptually. Presumably, all social theorists agree on these things, but such facts are not a sufficient basis from which to derive a social theory. Another fact about individuals is needed, a fact about behavioral motivations, such as innate selfishness or aggressiveness. But facts about motivations cannot be derived from facts about the biology we share with animals: Claims about such facts all depend upon further interpretations, which may seem convincing to some people in a particular time and place but which cannot be empirically demonstrated. That is, the "facts" about human nature that have traditionally provided any given social theory with its analytical power have been assumptions that the theorist derived from his or her own social values. The moral implications of an image of human nature have always been derived from a prior moral assumption sneaked into the image disguised as a fact.

In particular, these theories of human nature have generally ignored, or, rather, taken for granted, the concerns of
physical health—the physiology and biology of the body—as
essential contributors to the interests and needs of human
beings, that is, to human nature. It has been assumed that
whatever human nature is, it is not analytically related to
physiological processes as far as social theory is concerned.
Nothing critical about human motivations can be learned
from the determinants and conditions of individual physical
health. Social theorists have left the empirical and physiological facts of individual health to the physicians and medical biologists as essentially a separate and distinct aspect of
human life. Yet I believe that any serious analysis of human
life, of human nature, must include an understanding of the
physical as well as the social aspects of that life. In addition,
I believe that if it can be shown that health is both an empirical and a moral concern, then the integration of the
physiological and conceptual dimensions of human life into a
unified notion of human nature can provide the empirical
certainty and the moral direction for a demonstrably valid
analysis of human society. Such an analysis is what all social
theorists have sought, but by ignoring the concerns of physical health, all have had to introduce tacit moral assumptions
without an empirical base, thus making their theories products of cultural values rather than of empirical knowledge.

It should also be clear that, in spite of their ignoring the
issues of physical health, the social theorists have been fully
involved with the concerns of mental and social health. Any
conception of human nature is by implication a conception of
human health, for it indicates what individuals need, want,
and desire in order to be fully human, that is, in order
to be healthy humans. Any idea of what human beings really
are with respect to social motivations tells us what kind of
institutions and interactions they need in order to be socially

healthy. If they are naturally sociable and trusting, then they must be able to express that sociability and trust, or their health, indeed, their very humanity, will suffer. Accordingly, we need to build institutions that encourage community and trust, and such institutions can legitimately be judged as healthy. On the other hand, if humans are naturally aggressive, they must be allowed to express that aggression or their health will suffer. However, in this case there is a further problem, for by definition aggression on the part of one individual is a threat to the health of other individuals. In addition, it may be a threat to an individual's own health to the degree that his or her aggression threatens the stability of the social order, which is also a natural need. Here we need institutions that maximize individual aggression within the limits of social stability, and we must accept a certain amount of individual ill health, although such institutions themselves must be considered healthy.

Ideas about human nature entail ideas about individual and social health. As they have been traditionally formulated, though, these ideas only entail conclusions about mental health with respect to individuals. Moreover, as we have seen, the great tradition of social theory and social science has regarded human nature as fundamentally competitive, aggressive, and individualistic, naturally oriented toward the achievement of individual dominance through the inflicting of general pain and suffering. Undoubtedly, contemporary and historical evidence would seem to support this conception insofar as we are all aware of both subtle and grotesque instances of the mistreatment and destruction of some people by others. Yet the evidence is not conclusive at all. Indeed, even the nature of such evidence is uncertain with respect to whether these instances have been determined by the natural needs of all human beings to dominate and cause pain or by particular historical circumstances and cultural values that necessitate such acts but can be consciously changed, thus eliminating the need for such suffering. I have suggested that the general commitment to the former interpretation by modern social science rests on an unjustified moral assumption rather than a convincing demonstration. But such a commitment does exist and is supported by the view that human nature is in fundamental contradiction with itself insofar as it seems to demand individual actions that, taken as a whole, strongly conflict with the social conditions necessary for such actions to be possible.

From this view it follows that the basic requirements for human health are in conflict with themselves, that the concept of health itself, when applied to human beings, is logically incoherent. As we have seen, the health of an individual depends upon the attainment of essential personal control, mental and physical, moral and material. To the degree that the bases for conscious choice and effective action are incompatible, the effort to end the systematic human suffering caused by modern social institutions is not only practically but also logically impossible. If the very possibility of social life depends upon the systematic denial of essential human needs to at least some people, then social institutions must indeed make some people systematically ill if they are to maintain social order and social life. Since the achievement of healthy personal control by some necessitates the material and moral deprivation and unhealth of others, we can either guarantee equal access to material needs and protections—thus committing our institutions to unreservedly fostering physical health, with the consequence that everyone is denied the effective individual control, the individual freedom, that is required for moral health—or we can permit only some people to achieve that basic personal control—thus committing our institutions to protect that privileged access to health through the systematic and socially intended deprivation and unhealth of nearly everyone else. The former possibility (socialism) denies human health in the moral sense to everybody and therefore cannot be a human society, so we are left with the latter as the only "objective" possibility for the proper functioning of a society.

Thus, because individuals are fundamentally and naturally in conflict with their social life, a healthy society is one that systemically and purposefully makes many of its people sick. And since we recognize that, for all the scientific analysis, this conclusion still sounds a little odd, we commit many of our resources to a showy effort to cure illness (though it would be socially irresponsible to prevent illness entirely), we insist repeatedly that, formally at least, the ranks of the healthy few are open to all, and we find some solace in the claim that it is only the proportion of the healthy to the deprived, not the particular occupants of those categories, that must remain more or less constant. According to the assumptions of modern social science, the best society can only be the best compromise among competing human needs, and this compromise, as we have formulated and institutionalized it, fits nicely with the medical conception of human health, for it entails that our social institutions are so objectively healthy in their basic structure, regardless of the suffering they cause, that the only reasonable, the only professional, approach to the understanding and treatment of illness, injury, and breakdown is through the idea of the physiological and functional autonomy of the individual. That is, it follows from this approach to the analysis of social life that the judgment of health is indeed a technical, not a moral, judgment, for the criteria for the evaluation of social health are fundamentally different from, as well as opposed to, the criteria for the evaluation of individual health, and the determination of either depends solely upon the objective and scientific understanding of proper functioning. In both cases the judgment of health is a technical evaluation of necessary mechanisms rather than a moral critique of political power and economic decisions.

At this point it is important to remember the precise nature of the real society—our own—that we are discussing. It is neither an accident nor a natural necessity that we have a set of institutions whose proper working makes many people ill. Nor is it an accident that we have established and entrenched both a social theory and a medical theory that make these institutions seem reasonable and normal. Our capitalist society is a class society in the sense that there is a crucial difference between owners and nonowners, which is easily translated into the difference between the rich and the poor (with the famous middle class more and more falling into the latter group). One obvious consequence of this difference is that the rich few have enormous political and economic decision-making power while everyone else has very little, if any. Naturally, since being poor is an unpleasant prospect, the rich few are going to try to maintain their power and privilege at all costs, which means using their decision-making power to promote meaningless and alienating work, corrupt unions, racism, sexism, a largely unorganized work force, poor living conditions, poor transportation, a brutalizing police force, an unequal and property-biased legal system, and so on. But these are, of course, some of the systematic ways in which people are made ill. In other words, a capitalist economy such as ours depends upon a small but powerful class systematically fostering frustration and powerlessness, and therefore ill health, among a much larger class or classes. Furthermore, the class of owners and managers, in order to maintain their privilege, must maximize not only their control but also the profit of their corporations and enterprises, which means cutting costs, typically by disregarding the health and safety of the workers and by disregarding the health and safety of consumers with respect to products and the environment. These practices are common in our society, not because capitalists or managers willfully like to make people suffer, but because those who try to remedy these effects in their own businesses will necessarily lose profits and very likely lose their privileged position. In other words, our institutions demand that many people be made unhealthy as a conscious consequence of the systematic need to maintain class control and power, that the members of the working class, the service class, and the underclass of welfare recipients and unemployed be used, abused, and then effectively dismissed and discarded without their ever becoming fully aware of their own condition, much less organizing and acting to rectify it.

Of course, this effort to keep the powerless class from becoming fully aware and analytically conscious of their powerlessness is the role of ideology—with respect to the issues of this book, the role of social and medical theory. If my arguments are correct, the social scientific paradigm of inherent contradiction and the medical model of physiological functioning can only be understood as efforts to confuse and mislead, for purposes of social control, a class's understanding of itself and its society. Like the feudal theology of the Christians, the suffering of an oppressed class is interpreted as natural and inevitable, and the intuitive human sense that each of us has or should have a significant degree of control over the social and personal events in our lives is "scientifically," but categorically, denied, even to the extent of denying that our physical health, our physical body, is connected in any way with our personal consciousness, our social interaction, or our natural environment. As an analytical effort to understand human social life, these ideas are dismaying at the least, but as part of an ideological effort to maintain a controllable and malleable consciousness on the part of an oppressed and frustrated class, the institutional success and legitimacy of these ideas makes far more sense.

CHAPTER EIGHT

THE MORAL AND POLITICAL CERTAINTY OF HEALTH

Among the framers of modern social thought, only Marx envisioned that individual health and social health could be and should be compatible, and in this century only the followers of Marx have continued to develop and insist upon that possibility. Marx's idea of human health was severely limited—essentially, the absence of alienation and exploitation—and, like other social theorists, he simply assumed that it would be fully achieved in a society that functioned properly according to some objective social laws. More important, however, he did not accept systematic and institutionally generated human suffering as inevitable and try to justify it through an appeal to necessary and objective laws. Rather, he contended that social institutions need not discriminate against a major segment of the population in order to obey some higher scientific truth and that the people who are made sick by this discrimination need not accept their condition as the result of a tragic conflict in human nature, as the only way to avoid social disorder and anomic suicide, or as the price some must pay to live in a rational and efficient society. Such discrimination, he argued, is historical and cultural, not objective and necessary, and it can be completely eliminated through conscious political actions that would lead to a definitive improvement in human health, both physical and mental.

In the terms used here, Marx recognized that the concept

of health is not internally contradictory and that it is an inherently moral and political term. In accordance with the ordinary understanding, socially generated human unhealth (he uses such notions as alienation, reification, and the commodity exchange of labor) is something that should be politically and theoretically attacked, and the causes of unhealth should be eliminated. Thus, the judgment of individual health involves the judgment of social institutions, and if illness and breakdown are systemic in the society, then the judgment of health is a severe moral and political critique of those institutions, one that logically endorses change. Marx pointed out, and it should be apparent to all of us through the natural language, that social institutions that systematically destroy human health cannot be justified and that the effort to do so through the idea that the requirements for individual health are incompatible with the social achievement of individual health is logically contradictory and incoherent.

In his early writings, where he pays philosophical attention to such notions as alienation and species-being, Marx specifically denies what virtually all other social theorists affirm in one way or another: the idea that conflict is inherent in any relationship between individual and society, between consciousness and nature, or between individual and individual.

> My universal consciousness is only the *theoretical* form of that whose *living* form is the real community, the social entity, although at the present day this universal consciousness is an abstraction from real life and is opposed to it as an enemy. . . .
> It is above all necessary to avoid postulating "society" once again as an abstraction confronting the individual. The individual *is* the *social being*. The manifestation of his life—even when it does not appear directly in the form of a communal manifestation, accomplished in as-

> sociation with other men—is, therefore, a manifestation
> and affirmation of *social life.* . . . Though man is a
> unique individual—and it is just his particularity which
> makes him an individual, a real *individual* communal
> being—he is equally the *whole*, the ideal whole, the
> subjective existence of society as thought and experi-
> enced. He exists in reality as the representation and the
> real mind of social existence, and as the sum of human
> manifestations of thought. (Marx, p. 158, his emphasis)

Here Marx reiterates, in different formulations, his conviction that individual human beings are fully and integrally
social beings and thus cannot be in any sense inherently
antagonistic to society or to one another. But, of course, the
society in which he lived and wrote, capitalist society, produced mutually antagonistic individuals. This fact, which has
led all other theorists to postulate an intrinsic conflict, led
Marx to conclude that the institutions of capitalism, in particular wage (alienated) labor and private property, necessitate that individuals will face each other as hostile beings:
"*Private property* is thus derived from the analysis of the
concept of *alienated labor*; that is, alienated man, alienated
labor, alienated life, and estranged man" (p. 131, his emphasis). Rather than theoretically accepting the inevitability of
conflict and antagonism, with all the associated problems of
human health, Marx argued that we should replace capitalis-
tic institutions with ones that will encourage and strengthen
our natural social commitments instead of distorting and per-
verting them. In other words, Marx felt that we could act
consciously and politically to overcome the institutional
sources of conflict and oppression and thus the systematic
causes of ill health. The institutions to do this would be
those of a communistic society, according to Marx, and in
such a society all the allegedly inherent conflicts would be
resolved:

> *Communism* is the *positive* abolition of *private property*, of *human self-alienation*, and thus the real *appropriation* of *human* nature through and for man. It is therefore, the return of man himself as a *social*, i.e., really human, being, a complete and conscious return which assimilates all the wealth of previous development. Communism as a fully developed naturalism is humanism and as a fully developed humanism is naturalism. It is the *definitive* resolution of the antagonism between man and nature, and between man and man. It is the true solution of the conflict between existence and essence, between objectification and self-affirmation, between freedom and necessity, between individual and species. It is the solution to the riddle of history and knows itself to be this solution. (p. 155, his emphasis)

This is a glorious statement, and although it clearly makes my point about Marx vis-à-vis other social theorists, it also points to the problems of Marxist formulations and, indeed, to the similarities between Marx and rival social theorists. On the basis of his analysis of the capitalist forms of property and labor, Marx assumes that the good society, the one in which individuals are no longer in conflict with their social, or species, being, is the one in which private property, wage labor, and class power are no longer structurally possible. That is, human health—in his terms, the abolition of alienation, oppression, and mystification—will result from the dismantling of the system of private property, which is the basis for class power and class ideology. To his credit, Marx believed that individual health and social health are fundamentally compatible, even identical, but his idea of the components of this health and of the institutions to achieve it is no more analytically sound than the similar notions of the theorists already criticized. That is, Marx simply defines the good society, human health, in terms of the abolition of capitalist structures. As a result, he has no independent criteria by which to judge individual or social health.

For his argument about the good society to be convincing, Marx must hold an image of individual human health that is independent of his institutional-economic argument and then show that this latter argument envisions institutions that would create the conditions, according to the independent criteria, for individual and social health. As it stands, the Marxist argument leads easily to an assertion that a healthy society will result from the establishment of communistic institutions, an assertion that is at least historically doubtful and, indeed, has no claim to logical coherence. As I have argued, the concept of health is too powerful, too naturally meaningful, for any social theorist simply to appropriate it as part of his or her conceptual structure. Marx, of course, does not employ the term health as such, but he certainly implies its applicability; for example, he would never accept the idea that the communistic society is an unhealthy society. Without an independent means of judging the presence of human health, however, we have no more reason to believe that the abolition of private property will contribute to it than we do to believe that Freudian psychoanalysis or Durkheimian division of labor will do so.

I believe there are, in fact, independent reasons for agreeing with the Marxist claim over the others, but these reasons involve an understanding of the nature and requirements for human health, which Marx only vaguely and nonsystematically grasped. In particular, they involve a conceptualization of how healthy social relations, which Marx analyzed brilliantly at the theoretical level, cannot be logically separated from the empirical, and in an important sense nontheoretical, realities of the physical health of human beings, an issue that Marx and other social theorists fail to mention. Indeed, it is only by considering systematically the issue of physical health as an integral part of human, and thus of social, health that one can hope to develop an independent set of criteria for the establishment of a healthy society.

Like most other social theorists, Marx decided upon an image of what human beings are *really* like and then announced the discovery of objective laws that necessitate the building of institutions compatible with that human nature. If health were a more typical moral concept, on the order of freedom or justice—that is, one without an apparently straightforward empirical referent—Marx could simply define what he meant by it and proceed theoretically to construct a society that would provide it, as Mill did with respect to liberty and Plato and Rawls did with respect to justice. We might disagree with Mill about liberty or with Plato about justice, but this would be a disagreement about definitions, about values, and if their societies worked as they expected, they would not be compelled to agree with our critique. But we could disagree with Marx on an empirical basis about the health of the people in his society, and if we were right, he would be compelled to agree with us. It could not be simply a conflict of values, because health is uniquely a moral concept with an empirical referent. For many practical and theoretical purposes, the judgment of physical health—and even in some important ways the judgment of mental health—is in fact reasonably objective and noncontroversial.

The judgment of health, then, can provide a moral and political critique of social institutions and have a legitimate claim to empirical certainty. In its everyday usage it can and does bridge the gap between facts and values. It is no wonder, then, that an intense and rather successful medical and scientific effort has been made to deny the concept its moral status, to treat it as a technical term. One of the central aspects of this effort, the one to which Marx fell prey, has been to address the health of individuals *as* individuals solely from the perspective of physiological functioning (with occasional gestures toward social maladjustment) and to address the health of individuals *as* members of society, that is, the health of social institutions and of society, only with respect to the moral and productive aspects of social life—the fulfillment of psychological needs, the conditions of consciousness, and the production of the basic necessities for human life. From this separation has come the medical obsession with biology and the social scientific concentration on society as an organization or a system (of production, of values, and the like) and on the individual as a social element (a laborer, a taker of roles, a social actor, a believer in values, a bundle of instincts, a rational calculator, a symbolic self, etc.).

Yet human beings are all of these things—both biological and social, physiological and moral. We understand this naturally, though not very articulately, through the use of language, but we have forgotten it professionally and scientifically. Moreover, the concept of human health is not contradictory; the possibility of general social and biological well-being is not institutionally inconceivable. If we made more effort to remember this, to reconnect conceptually these separated components, it would affect both our practice of medicine and our practice of social analysis. In medicine, the doctors and their apologists would have to recognize the moral significance of health. To the degree that they were truly concerned with health, they would necessarily become participants in the evaluation and dismantling of institutions that generate human suffering. In the social sciences, analysis of the conditions and determinants of human health, particularly physiological health, would become a major theoretical concern, since these are major aspects of social life. Theorists could no longer simply define or assume what constitutes health by accepting an implicit or explicit conception of human nature; they would have to recognize the empirical aspects of health and our natural understanding of it. The underlying assumption of inherent contradiction would have to be brought into the open, discussed, and rejected if the concept of health were fully analyzed and integrated into social theory.

Together with an understanding of the conceptual unity and essential compatibility of social and physiological health, the analysis of institutions would have to include the inherently moral and empirically certain critique of their contribution to the conditions of human health. The institutional withholding or destruction of the basic requirements for human life and health for a major part of the population could no longer be either ignored or justified through insistence on the fundamental importance of moral health (as defined to mean some version of political freedom, such as the availability of the vote). In particular, institutions that generate poverty and malnutrition, that produce nutritionless and even harmful foods and then deny the availability of any other food, that structure transportation into the major cause of death and injury, that selectively deny the availability of essential health services, that treat individuals as less than human through racism, sexism, bureaucracy, and mindless work—institutions like these could not be judged as healthy. Also, institutions that systematically destroy the very conditions for all life and health—the air, water, and soil, the oceans, the forests, and the atmosphere—these institutions would have to be judged as extremely unhealthy. In other words, if the unity of physiological health and moral health were incorporated as a basic concept into social science, it would force an analysis of ecology into social theory, an understanding of the relations between production and the environment, between social life and natural processes. Moreover, because health is a moral issue, this understanding would be not only critical but also constructive: it would help us to rebuild and reorient our institutions toward the achievement of general human health through a recognition of its social, biological, and ecological aspects.

It is this understanding that has been missing from all social theory, including that of Marx, since it has not been theoretically accepted that human beings, as social participants, have a physiology and a biology and are practically, as well as conceptually, irrevocably a part of both the natural world and the social world. To the degree that natural processes have been introduced into social considerations, as in ethology and sociobiology, they have been regarded as conceptually prior to and strictly determinative of the social aspects of human life. Thus, even more than the doctors, these theorists simply deny the relevance of the moral concerns of human health, indeed, of all social life. It would seem, then, that through a more thorough analysis and acceptance of health as one of, if not the, central concept for an understanding of human life, we could begin to overcome some of the conceptual confusions and practical horrors that have been traditionally legitimated by our medical and social sciences.

Finally, the notion of health as a critical concept for the evaluation of social institutions has interesting implications. With respect to the judgment of human health, the uniquely human aspects of the criteria are the moral considerations, the concern with individual responsibility and personal control, with conscious choices and effective actions; but the most obviously universal and empirical aspects of the criteria are those we use to evaluate physiological functioning. The former give the concept of health its moral stature, and the latter give it its objective certainty. Traditionally we have separated these criteria, reserving the former for the social scientists and the latter for the doctors, a practice that has generated the widespread conviction that an inherent contradiction exists in the criteria at the level of social and moral life. And since some degree of moral suffering is thus inevitable, it has also been accepted, more by omission than commission, that a certain amount of physical suffering is also unavoidable: some people must be morally and physically deprived if others are to have personal control, that is, good health. Thus it has been accepted that at the social level, that is, for a population as a whole, a fundamental conflict exists between the requirements for moral health and the requirements for physical health, however compatible these requirements may be for particular individuals. But I have argued that this conflict does not exist, that the assumption itself is illogical because it denies the obvious and natural coherence of the concept of health, and that the achievement of general good health and of institutions that support it is not inconceivable. If I am correct, if human health in society is indeed a consistent and coherent idea, then it follows that, with respect to human beings, health is a concept that cannot meaningfully be reduced to the sum of two or more conceptually distinct concepts. In other words, the health of a human being is not the sum of his or her physical health and mental health, for the criteria for determining the state of either of these are not independent of the criteria for evaluating the other. As a result, an analysis of physiological functioning must be logically and conceptually incorporated into the study of individual involvement in a moral and social world and vice versa, though, given this understanding, each could, of course, be abstracted to some degree from the other when it is necessary for the analysis and treatment of particular situations.

Thus, the judgment of individual health is all of a piece. Consequently, the judgment of social health is also all of a piece. For institutions, as for individuals, moral health and physical health are compatible and interdependent; one cannot exist without the other, and if we are to create the general conditions for one, we will at the same time be creating the general conditions for the other. Here is the most interesting implication of the analysis of the judgment of health, for it would seem to follow that the moral critique of institutions can be moved out of the realm of relativistic values and the metaphysical discussion of human nature and into the realm of empirical certainty. Political debate in our society has been centered on differing and irreconcilable claims to have understood the *essential* meaning of such terms as freedom, justice, equality, objective truth, and the like. In each case the argument is that from this understanding certain institutions could be established that would then guarantee the best possible conditions for general moral health, from which would follow, it is implied, the maximum possible achievement of general physical health. But these claims to moral clarity based on an assumption about human nature are not and can never be universally convincing, since there is no logical, and certainly no political, necessity about any particular conception of human nature. If one conception is institutionalized and proves to be wrong—and there seem to be good arguments against each particular one—the consequences for human health could be, and in fact have often been, devastating.

Instead, we might start from the other end, that is, stop trying to maximize physical health by understanding and creating the conditions for moral health but, rather, attempt to maximize moral health by understanding and creating the conditions for general physical health. If we conclude from the analysis of the concept of health that moral health is a necessary concomitant of physical health, then the conceptual task would seem to be far easier and far more subject to agreement. For as we have seen, there is no meaningful and coherent way to divide the judgment of health into separate and independent realms: physical health, mental health, and social health are necessarily all of a piece. Like the two sides of a coin, they may be conceptually separable, but they are absolutely interdependent: what happens to one of them determines completely what happens to the others. Thus, establishing general physical health should in fact guarantee the establishment of general social health, in the fullest moral sense, and, of course, general physical health can be approached as a straightforward physiological concern, an objective issue categorically different from the deeply subjective issues of freedom and justice. Thus, as a fully social and political term, health has an empirical and objective quality that other moral terms do not, a quality that makes it perhaps our fundamental moral concept in terms of clarity and action.

If this is the case, what are its concrete implications? What would be the practical consequences for institutions and social life if we build a physically healthy society? With only the briefest consideration, certain consequences would seem apparent. First, it would mean a set of productive institutions that do not systematically pollute the life and health-sustaining environment in which the people of the society live. This requirement in itself would almost certainly necessitate a fundamental change in our economic approach to production, and, perhaps even more drastically, it would probably demand a completely different approach to technology, that is, a complete reevaluation of the conceptual validity of our scientific approach to nature and its processes. Second, it would mean that no individual or group of individuals would be able to make their lives better, in terms of social power, prestige, and wealth, by creating and maintaining conditions that make other individuals systematically

unhealthy. This, too, would obviously have profound implications about the nature of our economic system and the
availability of political power. Third, it would mean that
every individual in the society would have as a right full
access to whatever nourishment, sanitation, living conditions, and health care are necessary for a healthy life. This
would, among other things, eliminate the existence of poverty as we know it.

Finally, and perhaps most profoundly, the establishment
of general physical health, according to the analysis that has
been given, would require a society in which each individual
would have a sense of basic responsibility for and control
over his or her own life. Physical health, that is, has direct
social dimensions. People can and are being made ill not by
pollution, accidents, or poverty but simply by having lost
the sense of controlling their own lives. Correcting this systematic source of unhealth would probably have the most
overwhelming effect of all on our current approach to social
life and social institutions.

These theoretical positions are clearly dictated by a moral
commitment to a healthy society, and they directly imply
particular concrete actions with respect to changing social
institutions. Of course, the practical possibility of achieving
these changes remains a difficult and complex concern, involving a serious, sensitive, and dedicated effort at political
education and organization. Nonetheless, using the concept
of health as the basis for social analysis and political action
makes both the theoretical goals and the concrete tasks far
less dependent upon the subjective ambiguities inherent in
the nonfalsifiable assumptions about human life that have of
necessity supported the different theoretical approaches to
such moral issues as freedom, justice, and equality. Human
health is both a general good and an objective condition;
thus, as a moral value, it directly entails a commitment to

particular social institutions and practical political actions. For this reason it is a unique moral term, and as such it is clearly the best contender as the underlying value for any serious social analysis concerned with bettering the human condition.

Although the structure of a society based on human health would not be hard to imagine, and although most people would agree that such a society would be a physically healthy one, there will be disagreement over whether it could work, that is, whether people would accept it. And this is the moral question: Would the people in such a society be free? Would they have justice? Would they be able to achieve general moral health? Many would strongly doubt that a society primarily oriented toward creating the conditions for universal *physical* health could ever be a morally acceptable, politically responsive context for human life. Yet, according to the argument I have presented, it would of necessity be such a society, for moral health and physical health are conceptually, and thus practically, inseparable. As concepts they refer to different perspectives of the same thing: human health. They are not independent; there are no separate criteria, and the existence of one logically implies the existence of the other. Thus, if general physical health were assured, general moral health would also be assured, and the conditions of physical health, unlike the conditions of moral health, can be empirically and objectively understood. This, then, would seem to make the task of achieving social health, of building the good society, somewhat easier and more straightforward.

Moreover, the unity of physical health and moral health presents a final solution to the relation between moral concepts and scientific knowledge. The society I envision would be one based on the achievement of health in its fullest and logical sense. Traditionally, social theorists have envisioned society based on such qualities as freedom, justice, equality, reason, happiness, order, and the like. These have commonly been seen as moral concerns in a sense that health is not, but in any case they are certainly worthwhile concerns and should be considered as relevant to considerations of any possible society. Assuming that we can build a society that is healthy, how can we be sure that it will also be free, just, and equal? And if we cannot be sure, which of these concerns should we take as our main priority? From the preceding analysis of the concept of health I believe it is clear that these problems cannot logically arise. Other moral concerns can only be synonyms for health in the sense that they mean essentially the same thing. More exactly, they would be synecdoches for health—parts that stand for the whole—so that freedom, justice, and equality would all be necessary contributors to the general condition of health. If this were not the case, we would be in a position of saying that a free society or a just society could be systematically unhealthy for some of its members, and for those individuals at least such a society would be neither free nor just.

In *A Healthy State*, Victor and Ruth Sidel write:

> Health care and medical care, like other services, are a means to an end, rather than an end in themselves. What then are *our* views on the ends of a health-care and medical-care system? What are *our* answers to the questions "For whom?" and "To what purpose?"
>
> 1. We believe that the most fundamental purpose of social institutions is that of justice—justice in its Aristotelian sense: a fair distribution of all that is of value in society. (Sidel and Sidel, p. xxv)

The Sidels are radicals with respect to their analysis of the problems of health, and they share with me the conviction that American institutions are systematically unhealthy and need to be changed. But I believe that this passage reveals a conceptual confusion that they share with many other radicals, as well as with far less radical doctors, philosophers, and social theorists. They claim that they can discuss health and health services technically but that they must independently establish the moral goals toward which those techniques should be directed. Further, they imply that the best they can do is to indicate their personal preference for those goals, that the moral direction of health techniques can only finally be a matter of personal choice and cultural values, and that justice is a legitimate, though finally arbitrary, direction in a sense that health is not.

As we have seen, however, this conclusion cannot be true of health. The desire to achieve health is not independent of the desire to achieve justice, and vice versa. It must be the case that the just society is the healthy society, the free society is the healthy society, the equal society is the healthy society, and so on. Indeed, it must even be the case that the just society is the *physically* healthy society, the free society is the *physically* healthy society, since physical health is not an independent aspect of social or mental health but is only a particular perspective on the general and unified condition of human health. Freedom, justice, health, and equality are all interdependent, but only health among them all has a solid and definitive empirical referent. Thus, moral terms such as freedom and justice must be defined in terms of health, for otherwise they are left free-floating, as the Sidels and most social theorists seem to think. When the concept of health is properly, that is, consistently, understood, the idea of a healthy society provides its own logically intrinsic goals, and those goals necessarily include such traditional concerns as freedom, justice, and equality.

The unifying idea of such a society, and thus of all these moral concerns, is that it makes no sense for a society as a whole to commit itself to moral goals whose achievement requires the systematic illness, injury, and death of some, many, or all of its members. It might make sense for a certain class or ruling group to try to convince the entire population that such goals are reasonable, but that is not the same thing. The healthy society is also free and just because it enables everyone—and that includes not only the present population but the future populations as well—be maximally healthy, that is, fully human. It excludes all institutions that force some people to be oppressed by—that is, made sick by—others, and it excludes any institution or technology that would in any way harm or disrupt the ecological system on which all life, and thus health, depend. The health of some cannot be achieved at the expense of the health of others, present or future. The necessary political systems, institutions, and technologies are those that fit naturally and nondisruptively into the encompassing ecology, insofar as the conception of that ecology is expanded to include the requirements for human health. But human health requires that each individual be able to make conscious choices and take effective actions, so that our supporting ecology cannot be conceived of as a biological system but rather as a system that ensures the achievement of both conscious and physical personal control by each individual. In other words, our human health, and thus our social structures and institutions, are integrally a part of that encompassing ecology we must not distort. Obviously, if we do distort it, our health will suffer. What has not been so obvious is that if we build a society with institutions and technologies that will not distort it, according to straightforward biological criteria, then our general health, both as individuals and as a society, will benefit, as will our relation to such concerns as freedom, justice, and equality.

This is the final point of the argument. Health is a concern

not only of our bodies and our societies but also of our
ecological system, which includes human society and social
institutions as part of its crucial components. All of these
must be healthy if we are to be healthy, and if the health of
any one of them is systematically threatened, then the health
of all is equally threatened. Human beings—conscious, effective human beings—as well as social institutions are inherently a part of the ecology of human life. A healthy ecology cannot be a simple biological problem, for a biologically
balanced ecology is clearly compatible with a great deal of
human oppression and suffering; indeed, it may be most
compatible with the elimination of the human race from that
system, provided that end is not achieved in certain ways. A
healthy ecology that includes human beings is a concern not
only of biology but also of societies, technologies, and the
possibility of individual consciousness. As the full implications of the concept of health are uncovered, they will suggest in increasing detail the kind of social institutions that
we must *choose* to establish in order to provide ecological
health as well as general individual health for human beings.
These institutions will be correctly considered healthy, for
they will make the concept of health consistent in all of its
uses and ensure that we are not destroying ourselves and
others by systematically turning one moral concern against
another. And we shall also see that these are the only institutions compatible with the biology of our bodies and our
natural environment, so that they are the ones morally entailed by the empirical determinants of health. The doctors
and social theorists notwithstanding, the judgment of health
is as decisively political as it is universal and scientific.

THE SIGNIFICANCE OF CONCEPTS

Health is a key aspect of human life and therefore should be a key concept for understanding that life. Curiously, however, the scientists and philosophers who have studied and theorized about human social life have generally ignored it as a subject for serious analysis. I have argued that when it is properly understood as a necessary moral concept, it logically entails an empirically certain critique of modern society and a definitive direction for political and economic change. It is a concept that is constitutive of human life itself, and since that life is both natural and social, both biological and moral, it is clear that this concept must decisively inform all of these spheres of activities. Empirically, it demands universal obligation; morally, it demands a principled commitment to constructing institutions and values compatible with human health.

To social and medical theorists, however, the concept is a technical one that refers to a scientific judgment about objective, neutral, and mechanical processes, primarily physiological ones. In particular, health is a concern of the biological individual's existence as a part of nature, that is, as a part of the mechanistic logic of natural laws. Such things as institutions, roles, production, and values are a part of the mechanisms of society, and such things as justice, freedom, equality, friendship, and dignity are part of the ambiguous, relativistic, probably overstated, and certainly nonscientific realm of human consciousness, purpose, and commitment. As individuals, we are continuously involved in these latter things, particularly the mechanisms of society, but, according to the doctors, such things have little if anything to do with our health. As we have come to understand it medically, health is an attribute of an individual's biology and physiology, which human beings share equally and technically with all other forms of life.

To the degree that this medical view is in fundamental conflict with our natural understanding of health, it raises a further question: Why are there two competing sets of criteria available for understanding the concept of health? If there is a natural understanding inherent in the concept itself, why is the medical understanding not aligned with it? Why do the doctors insist that health is something completely technical, objective, and physiological? If these two ideas of health are so decisively exclusive of one another that serious practical and conceptual confusion has resulted, there must be some reason this mess has occurred.

Very briefly, we can trace the beginnings of this dilemma to the metaphysical, even ideological, attitudes and perspectives underlying the rise of modern science, namely, the acceptance of what we have come to know as the mind-body dualism. Before the rise of science, and the concomitant rise of capitalism, virtually all societies were organized on the basis of religious institutions and political traditions, and health was generally understood as involving not only the mechanisms of the body but also such things as personal intention, interpersonal hostility, moral responsibility, and social obligations. At the beginning of the modern age, the mathematical and mechanistic ideas of Kepler, Galileo, and Newton were decisively instrumental in breaking both the intellectual and moral authority of the Church and thus in legitimating a new form of class power, economic production, and personal relationships—a new social order.

First Hobbes and Descartes, and then all subsequent

social theorists and moral philosophers, used the scientific approach to nature as a basis for describing and analyzing social life and human interaction. Hobbes in particular decided that social life could be understood in terms of the same mechanistic analysis of motions that Galileo was imposing upon nature, only in this case the essential motions became the fundamental and rational desire of every individual for accumulation and self-interest, and the mechanism became universal competition. All traditional authorities and obligations were rejected; social life could be completely reduced to the rational decisions of autonomous, self-interested individuals. Concurrently, Descartes used the same scientific reasoning to argue that human beings are materially a part of nature and therefore subject to the same deterministic, mechanical laws that govern all matter.

Yet human beings also have consciousness, that is, a sense of intention, purpose, and responsibility, which are theoretically incompatible with the fundamental certainty of the mechanistic determinism of nature. Thus, as far as human beings are concerned, there must be two realms: the physical realm of the body, where everything is determined and all actions and events follow precise, immutable, and mathematical laws, and the conscious realm of the mind, where it is possible to have a conscious understanding of our physical imprisonment and thus to become truly, but only mentally, free. Physically, we are like everything else in nature; nonetheless, our true humanity, our sense of choice, purpose, and responsibility, is real enough so long as we accept that it is exclusively a mental, and not a physical, reality. Thus the mind was split off from the body and the central core of human experience as such was relegated to an ephemeral and detached consciousness of that experience. In combination these ideas produced the metaphysical perspective of most modern social thought: both the body and society are governed by mechanical, natural laws, whereas the characteristically human activities—consciousness and choice—are decisively separate from both, existing only, but importantly, in the isolated minds of autonomous individuals.

It is not hard to see the consequences of such an idea for the understanding of health. So far as treatment and social organization are concerned, health must necessarily become a function of the mechanical, that is physiological, order of the body. The crucial, consciousness-related aspects of human life have become so individualized and self-reflective that they can only be the subject of individual and theoretical, essentially philosophical, concern. They are, indeed, matters for the individual to contemplate, not an issue for the practical and serious analysis of health. With consciousness thus so severely individualized, the social aspects of human life, and thus of health, became interestingly problematic. For Hobbes and the early political theorists of capitalism, as well as for Adam Smith and the more recent economic theorists of capitalism, society is basically only a concatenation of individuals, so that the problem of society is only the problem of individual drives and interests. Such an approach leads directly back to those natural emotions and laws, to the idea of an inherent and substantive human nature. But although this idea seems to have remained acceptable, or at least necessary, for the theoretical defense of capitalist economics, it was too obviously simplistic to account for the enormous complexity of an industrializing civilization. It was an extreme idea that was immensely effective in the intellectual struggles against the traditions of feudalism, but as a basis for analyzing social life it was grossly inadequate.

The basic conception of social life inherent in this individualistic analysis nevertheless survived and came to dominate social thought. The great social theorists of the last century, particularly Durkheim, believed that society is not a simple concatenation of individuals but rather an independent and autonomous reality, one that cannot be analytically reduced to individual interests. This reality, however, also follows natural, preordained laws, just as do nature and its processes, and these laws, like the laws of nature, are discoverable through the scientific method and are inherent and immutable. We can learn them and endlessly refine our knowledge of them, but we cannot change them. Once again we are characterized by our ability to have consciousness of our world and our lives, but we must accept that consciousness as both self-defining and ineffective; it can only be a consciousness of our fate.

As we have seen, this was an old idea. The new insight, which laid the foundation for modern social science, was that these laws of society are of an order essentially different from that of the laws of nature. The study of society falls within the general scientific framework of acquiring knowledge, but this study has its own unique logic, concepts, and methods. So now there are two fundamental and scientific dimensions: society is a thing-in-itself and nature is a thing-in-itself. Human beings are a part of both, but in either dimension their lives and actions are governed by precise and deterministic laws and mechanisms. A third dimension, consciousness, establishes the essential freedom and humanity of human beings, but it is ineffective, practically irrelevant, and completely nonscientific. Consciousness is individualized and discounted, and human beings are doubly determined—by their society with respect to social interaction and by nature with respect to their bodies.

The fundamental consequences for the notion of health implied by this new idea of the autonomous reality of society were not immediately apparent. The pervasive idea that the individual's essential existence is autonomous, not social, and that our practical existence is mechanistically physical rather than purposeful and intentional was leading the theorists and practitioners of health more and more in the direction of a biological definition. With the new view of society, it appeared conceivable for society to break down in the same sense that the body breaks down, and consequently the idea of social health was fleetingly discussed. But, given the conception of the autonomy and regularity of society, this was too much like discussing the health of gravity or the health of an atom, and this direction for incorporating the social aspects of life, based upon the new social scientific idea of society, into the analysis of health proved fruitless.

But a new direction soon emerged, one that has proved infinitely fruitful and has added a decisive new ingredient into the modern discussion of health. This was the direction of Freud and the development of the notion of mental health. Freud recognized that the scientifically accepted notion of two autonomous realities, nature and society, could be interpreted as leaving individual human beings in something of a bind. Since both nature and society have their own independent mechanisms, it could be that those mechanisms are in fundamental conflict, in which case each individual will necessarily be in fundamental self-conflict. The demands of society will in some way inevitably contradict the demands of nature. Freud developed this idea brilliantly, taking the individualistic notion of our essentially physical, self-interested, and competitive natural existence and running it smack up against the social demands of group cohesion. The result, according to Freud and his followers, is mental breakdown, the idea that our consciousness will be distorted to the point that we can no longer carry on normal and effective social lives. Here the dimensions both of society and of consciousness are brought back into the discussion of health. Significantly, however, it is a detached

discussion of health: mental health is not connected with
physical health, consciousness is still detached from the body.
Moreover, it is not consciousness in the sense of the characteristic human activities of choice and purpose. Rather, it is
consciousness in the sense of a negotiation between the opposing forces of nature and society, between independent
and powerful determinations. Consciousness becomes a way
of getting our mechanisms together; it remains a way of
reconciling ourselves to our deterministic fate. Society is an
independently existing threat to health when it forces us to
repress our natural desires. Nature is also guilty when it
demands that we defy the necessary social order. Mental
health consists of adjusting our individual needs and drives
to the requirements of society, just as physical health consists of adjusting our physical activities to the mechanisms of
the body. Mental health, then, like physical health, is an
individual, technical, and objective concern. Both society
and nature are objective and immutable, and the individual
consciousness must be adjusted to their demands. This is a
technical procedure, and the knowledge of it, like the knowledge of nature and society, is objective.

When Freud brought consciousness finally into the scientific fold, the mind-body split was in some sense closed.
But it is a pyrrhic closure, for the basic concern of Descartes, Kant, Sartre, and others with the experienced reality
of human freedom, human choice, and human purpose is
not included; indeed, in some sense these concerns are no
longer seen as even an aspect of consciousness. Freud's way
of bringing consciousness and society into the discussion of
health leaves the basic physical definition of health unaffected. Mental health is defined as completely separate from
physical health; moreover, it is defined exactly on the model
of physical health. Both are absolutely individual and objective concerns, which, when understood properly, raise none

of the moral and political issues involved with the direction, quality, and purpose of human life. If the basic criteria for the evaluation of mental health are not the same as the criteria for physical health, they are nevertheless of the same type, and both sets of criteria will conflict necessarily with any natural understanding of health as a concept that characterizes the full and unique potential of human life. As a matter of fact, through the efforts of the behavioralists and others, the criteria for the evaluation of mental health are becoming more and more aligned with the criteria for physical health as human consciousness is redefined in such a way that it can be scientifically reduced to physiological processes.

This, of course, is the logical extension of the original scientific view of nature, the mind-body dualism, and the individualized view of human beings and health. In a world governed by the autonomous laws of nature, of society, of economics, and now of technology, human consciousness, like the feudal God of the Christians, becomes irrelevant, and human control over the direction and processes of social life becomes theoretically, at least, inconceivable, a satisfying fantasy for the nonscientific. The medical view of health is the logical consequence of such a perspective, such a society. As a theory, I have argued, it conflicts decisively with our natural understanding of health, but as an *ideology* it corresponds exactly with the commitments of our modern technological society to elite, technical control, to class power, to technical development and profit as ends in themselves, and to the systematic, bureaucratic dehumanization of human life. It is for this reason—class dominance and ideological control—that the medical perspective has established such a decisive monopoly upon our thinking about human health.

It would seem apparent that this perspective cannot establish its view definitively, despite its ideological connections with social power and its real biological successes. For, as I have suggested, it will inevitably run afoul of our necessary sense that human life and human health must consist of much more than this kind of medicine and this kind of social life permit. But there is another problem here. The medical attitude toward health has rendered the very idea of life itself increasingly problematic. To say that something or someone is biologically alive is no longer the same as saying that the thing or person is alive as the term is ordinarily used in the natural language. The obvious example is the case where an individual's brain has been damaged or destroyed but the body is being kept "alive"—in the sense that the organs are still functioning, the blood is still circulating—by machines in a hospital. In such a case we have a hard time referring to this person as in any normal sense "alive." Since we must, both because the definition of life is no longer in the public domain and because in some few cases recovery from such a condition is possible, we have begun to rely on a new, more compatible way of referring to such people in ordinary conversation: we often say that people in that condition have become "vegetables." Used in this way, the term clearly indicates that we must find new conceptual ways to distinguish the condition of life from the condition of human life: being a living human being is no longer necessarily the same thing as having human life. Since health is an evaluation of the quality of human life, there is now a point at which "living" for a human being can no longer be meaningfully qualified by the concept of health used in the normal way. As a result, the very nature of the being itself must be conceptually redefined.

This subtle change in our understanding of human life and human health has been made necessary by the technical theories and advances of modern medicine. "Life" has become a technical condition of biological functioning. Another interesting example of this conceptual change—and a crucial one considering the stunning environmental and political dangers of recombinant DNA—is the way research biologists have solved both the problem of vitalism and the problem of the origin of life by simply redefining life as a chemical, and therefore mechanical, process. Clearly, modern medicine is having a significant effect on the ways in which we think about ourselves and our lives, as well as upon the technology, and thus the institutions, of our society. Moreover, as opposed to the medical version of health, which can be strongly, even empirically, critiqued as fundamentally wrong with respect to a more natural and universal understanding, the medical version of life is more convincing. To oppose it on the grounds of a more natural understanding would mean to argue, for example, for the evaluation of the "human vegetables" as being no longer really alive, an evaluation whose logical consequences, since recovery is sometimes possible, could be strongly attacked on at least some humanitarian grounds. Through its ability to redefine technically much of our natural understanding of human life, scientific medicine obviously has been able to save many lives that would otherwise have been lost. Thus, the problem of the concept of life may be even more complex than the problem of the concept of health, for it would seem at first glance that the two versions of life may be more fundamentally contradictory than the two versions of health.

The obvious question, of course, is why would anyone think that the concept of life presents any problem at all. That the medical and biological definition of life makes it possible for us to save more lives and to prolong life in some cases should be prima facie evidence of the inherent merit and value of this definition. The problem, though, is that the kind of life that biology may prolong and the kind of life that most of us are in favor of may not be at all the same thing. Remember that the very concept of life itself is being changed and redefined; that is, the term itself may mean different things with respect to different contexts and different people. We are in favor of a life that allows us to some degree at least to be human, with all that implies about conscious control and effective actions. Yet the life that the biologists talk about is a strictly chemical and physiological one. As Nobel Prize–winning biochemist Jacques Monod puts it, "Living beings are chemical machines" (Monod, p. 45). S. E. Luria, another biologist and Nobel laureate, concurs:

> Life in action is the functioning of living organisms, the molecular and atomic events brought about by the presence of life, and is the subject matter of biochemistry. . . . To the scientist, the uniqueness of man is purely a biological uniqueness. . . . (Luria, pp. 5, 7)

With respect to cases of brain damage, the human vegetables, this difference in definition may not seem important; indeed, it may seem generally beneficial. But these are the unequivocal showcases of medical and scientific understanding. As the concept of life becomes increasingly biological, technical, and given over to experts, many other applications and effects are possible and are in fact already present. A prime example is the use of drugs to lower human consciousness and participation while adequately maintaining biological life. Many thousands of people, from housewives to prisoners, from children to the aged, are already kept in a more or less permanently drugged condition in order to make their consciousness compatible with their social role. And it may well be possible in the future to keep entire racial or sexual groups—indeed, entire classes or nations—in a constant drug-induced stupor (one compatible, of course, with certain menial and routine tasks and functions) so that they will not challenge and never even fully understand their manipulation and dominance by others. At what point, then, is such a drugged life compatible with human life? Must we find a new term, such as human vegetables, for these people also, or is their drug-induced "life" the same as that of the drug givers? At what point does a "living," that is, biologically functioning, member of the human species stop being a human being as we normally understand the term? Before the medical-scientific redefinition of life, such a question would have been impossible, a contradiction in terms. Now it is one of the crucial questions of our time, and it can only be answered so long as the concept of "life" retains its nontechnical, critical, and therefore moral meaning.

Perhaps an even more stunning, though we can hope less imminent, consequence of the biological version of life is the theoretical possibility of creating people by design through genetic engineering. Is someone (or something) who has been genetically programmed by scientists to have certain characteristics and abilities really a "human being"? The reaction of most of us is to think of such beings as either a joke or as some kind of robotlike machine. But how long will this reaction last in the face of the reality?

The real question, of course, is what does it mean to be a human being, to have human life, to experience human health? All our notions of social life and our commitments to social values depend upon the answer to this question. I have argued that the answer is inherent in our ability to use language, to communicate conceptually, to direct our own lives consciously, and thus to produce ourselves through our actions. The answer is not culturally relative, arbitrary, or neutrally technical: it is a necessarily moral aspect of our human existence. Yet our natural understanding of our own human experience is being systematically and authoritatively discounted by scientists as an anthropocentric fantasy and definitively replaced by the "objective" ideas of science and medicine, ideas that achieve their dominant strength not through empirical and logical reasoning but rather through technical and ideological power, through the demands and distortions of class control. As we have seen, an impressive edifice of ideological understanding, from social theory to biology, has been constructed to defend the institutions and techniques of class power, with all their attendant poverty, oppression, ill health, and dehumanization. These institutions and techniques must be replaced by ones more compatible with human, and therefore with social and natural, life.

As I have tried to make clear, one of the initial and crucial elements of any fundamental reorganization of society must be to the recovery of the necessary meanings of the concepts that define and constitute our experience, our lives, and our health as human beings. Without an analytically clear and confident commitment to these concepts, our values will be relative and problematic and our actions either tentative or dogmatic. We cannot hope to know the positive direction for human life and human health if we do not fully understand what these terms mean. The authoritative power of medicine and, behind it, much of social and natural science have attempted to confuse us about these meanings in order to convince us that their technical definitions are the objectively correct ones, thus making these definitions both fundamentally ideological and conceptually oppressive. The power to change the basic concepts with which people understand themselves is the power to change the world in which those people live, and in this case it has been the power to transform inherently moral and political decisions concerning health, life, the social order, and the natural environment into technical decisions that are therefore best left to the experts and specialists of class privilege and control. This is the power we are increasingly giving to medical science and its supporting theories—the power to make the people in our society believe that, with respect to life and health, they are more mechanical than human, they are something less than people. It is an awesome power, perhaps the most awesome, for if it is fully realized, it will indeed succeed in turning many of us into something less than human—all in the name of health. It is the power inherent in the social definitions of concepts and their meanings, the power to control consciousness and understanding. We can only hope that a fuller realization of the nature of this power will make us more aware of the necessary meanings of these terms for human beings and therefore make us more resistant to the confiscation and misuse of such basic ideas as the notion of human health.

BIBLIOGRAPHY

Alford, Robert R. *Health Care Politics: Ideological and Interest Group Barriers to Reform*. Chicago: University of Chicago Press, 1975.

Ardrey, Robert. *The Social Contract: A Personal Inquiry into the Evolutionary Sources of Order and Disorder*. New York: Atheneum, 1975.

Aronson, Elliot. *The Social Animal*. New York: Random House, Vintage Books, 1972.

Barash, David P. *Sociobiology and Behavior*. New York: Elsevier North-Holland, Inc., 1977.

Bradley, John M. "Implications and Applications of Historical Materialist Epidemiology." In "HMO Packet #2: The Social Etiology of Disease (Part II), Implications and Applications of HME" (mimeographed), 1977.

Burns, Chester R. "Diseases vs. Healths: Some Legacies in the Philosophies of Modern Medical Science." In Engelhardt and Spiker, eds., *Evaluation and Explanation*, 1975, pp. 29–47.

———. "The Non-Naturals: A Paradox in the Western Concept of Health." *Journal of Medicine and Philosophy* 1, no. 3 (1976), 202–211.

Carlson, Rick. *The End of Medicine*. New York: John Wiley & Sons, 1975.

Churchill, Larry R. "Bioethical Reductionism and Our Sense of the Human." *Man and Medicine* 5, no. 4 (1980), 229–242.

Collins, Randall. *Conflict Sociology: Toward an Explanatory Science*. New York: Academic Press, 1975.

Concerned Rush Students. "Turning Prescriptions into Profits." *Science for the People* 9 (Jan.–Feb. 1977), 6–9, 30–32.

Daniels, Norman, ed. *Reading Rawls: Critical Studies on Rawls' "A Theory of Justice."* New York: Basic Books, 1975.

Dawkins, Richard. *The Selfish Gene*. New York: Oxford University Press, 1976.

Doyal, Lesley. *The Political Economy of Health*. Boston: South End Press, 1981.

Dubos, René. *Man, Medicine, and Environment*. New York: Mentor Book, New American Library, 1968.

Durkheim, Emile. *Suicide: A Study in Sociology*. Translated by John A. Spaulding and George Simpson. Edited by George Simpson. New York: Free Press, 1951.

————. *The Division of Labor in Society*. Translated by George Simpson. New York: Free Press, 1964.

————. *The Elementary Forms of the Religious Life*. Translated by Joseph Ward Swain. New York: Free Press, 1965.

Dworkin, Gerald. "Non-Neutral Principles." In Daniels, ed., *Reading Rawls*, 1975, pp. 124–140.

Ehrenreich, Barbara, and English, Deirdre. *For Her Own Good: 150 Years of the Experts' Advice to Women*. New York: Doubleday, Anchor Books, 1979.

Engel, George L. "The Biomedical Model: A Procrustean Bed?" *Man and Medicine* 4, no. 4 (1979), 257–275.

Engelhardt, H. Tristram, Jr. "Concepts of Health and Disease." In Engelhardt and Spiker, eds., *Evaluation and Explanation*, 1975, pp. 125–141.

Engelhardt, H. Tristram, Jr., and Spiker, Stuart, eds. *Evaluation and Explanation in the Biomedical Sciences*. Dordrecht: Reidel, 1975.

Eyer, Joseph. "Hypertension as a Disease of Modern Society." *International Journal of Health Services* 5, no. 4 (1975), 539–558.

Eysenck, Hans J. "Learning Therapy and Behavior Therapy." In Millon, ed., *Theories*, 1973, pp. 388–402.

Fabrega, Horacio, Jr., and Silver, Daniel B. *Illness and Shaministic Curing in Zinacantan*. Stanford: Stanford University Press, 1973.

Fisk, Milton. "History and Reason in Rawls' Moral Theory." In Daniels, ed., *Reading Rawls*, 1975, pp. 53–80.

Foot, Philippa. "Moral Beliefs." In Philippa Foot, *Virtues and*

Vices and Other Essays in Moral Philosophy, pp. 110–131. Berkeley: University of California Press, 1978.

Freud, Sigmund. *A General Selection from the Works of Sigmund Freud*. Edited by John Richman, M.D. New York: Doubleday and Co., 1957.

————. *Civilization and Its Discontent*. Edited and translated by James Strachey. New York: W. W. Norton and Co., 1961.

Gordon, Milton M. *Human Nature, Class, and Ethnicity*. New York: Oxford University Press, 1978.

Gorovitz, S. "Bioethics and Social Responsibility." In T. L. Beauchamp and L. Walters, eds., *Contemporary Issues in Bioethics*, pp. 52–60. Encino, Calif.: Dickenson Publishing Co., 1978.

Greenstein, Robert. "An End to Persistent Poverty and Hunger in America." In Lerza and Jacobson, eds., *Food for People*, 1975, pp. 311–319.

Hare, R. M. *The Language of Morals*. London: Oxford University Press, 1964.

————. *Essays on Philosophical Method*. London: Macmillan & Co., 1971.

————. "Rawls' Theory of Justice." In Daniels, ed., *Reading Rawls*, 1975, pp. 81–107.

Hart, H. L. A. "Rawls on Liberty and Its Priority." In Daniels, ed., *Reading Rawls*, 1975, pp. 230–252.

Hartmann, Heinz. "Psychoanalysis as a Scientific Theory." In Millon, ed., *Theories*, 1973, pp. 152–164.

Heath, Joe. "Genocide of the Mind." *Science for the People* 6 (May 1974), 8–15.

Himwich, Harold. "Psychopharmacologic Drugs." In Millon, ed., *Theories*, 1973, pp. 87–110.

Hobbes, Thomas. *Leviathan*. New York: Bobbs-Merrill, 1958.

Horton, Robin. "African Traditional Thought and Western Science." In B. Wilson, ed., *Rationality*, pp. 131–171. Oxford: Basil Blackwell, 1970.

Hughes, Richard, and Brewin, Robert. *The Tranquilizing of America*. New York: Harcourt Brace Jovanovich, 1979.

Hurley, Roger, ed. *Poverty and Mental Retardation: A Causal Relationship*. New York: Random House, Vintage Books, 1969.

Illich, Ivan. *Medical Nemesis: The Expropriation of Health*. New York: Pantheon, 1976.

Kety, Seymour. "Biochemical Hypothesis of Schizophrenia." In Millon, ed., *Theories*, 1973, pp. 118–138.

Lenski, Gerhard. *Power and Privilege: A Theory of Social Stratification*. New York: McGraw-Hill, 1966.

Lerza, Catherine, and Jacobson, Michael, eds. *Food for People, Not for Profit*. New York: Ballantine Books, 1975.

Lipset, Seymour Martin. "Value Patterns, Class and the Democratic Party: The United States and Great Britain." In R. Bendix and S. M. Lipset, eds., *Class, Status and Power*, pp. 161–171. New York: Free Press, 1966.

Lorenz, Konrad. *On Aggression*. Translated by Marjorie Kerr Wilson. New York: Harcourt Brace & World, Inc., 1966.

Luria, S. E. *Life: The Unfinished Experiment*. New York: Charles Scribner's Sons, 1973.

McCarthy, Colman. "Bon Chemical Appétit." In Lerza and Jacobson, eds., *Food for People*, 1975, pp. 57–64.

McKeown, Thomas. *The Role of Medicine*. London: Nuffield Provincial Hospitals Trust, 1976.

Maclean, Una. "Choices of Treatment among the Yoruba." In Morley and Wallis, eds., *Culture and Curing*, 1979, pp. 152–167.

Marx, Karl. *Early Writings*. Edited and translated by T. A. Bottomore. New York: McGraw-Hill, 1963.

Mill, John Stuart, and Bentham, Jeremy. *The Utilitarians: An Introduction to the Principles of Morals and Legislation*. Garden City, N.Y.: Doubleday, Anchor Books, 1973.

Millon, Theodore, ed. *Theories of Psychopathology and Personality*. Philadelphia: W. B. Saunders Co., 1973.

Monod, Jacques. *Chance and Necessity*. New York: Random House, Vintage Books, 1972.

Morley, Peter. "Culture and the Cognitive World of Traditional Medical Beliefs: Some Preliminary Considerations." In Morley and Wallis, eds., *Culture and Curing*, 1979, pp. 1–18.

Morley, Peter, and Wallis, Roy, eds. *Culture and Curing: Anthropological Perspectives on Traditional Medical Beliefs and Practices*. Pittsburgh: University of Pittsburgh Press, 1979.

Murphy, Edmond A. *The Logic of Medicine*. Baltimore: Johns Hopkins University Press, 1976.

Nagel, Thomas. "Rawls on Justice." In Daniels, ed., *Reading Rawls*, 1975, pp. 1–16.

Navarro, Vincente. *Medicine under Capitalism*. New York: Prodist, 1976.

Newton, Lisa. "Some Reflections on Political Nature: Conservative Theory Revisited." *Journal of Philosophy* 72 (Oct. 23, 1975), 593–604.

Parsons, Talcott. *The Social System*. Glencoe, Ill.: Free Press, 1964.

Pellegrino, Edmund, and Thomasma, David. *A Philosophical Basis of Medical Practice: Toward a Philosophy and Ethic of the Healing Professions*. New York: Oxford University Press, 1981.

Rawls, John. *A Theory of Justice*. Cambridge, Mass.: Harvard University Press, 1971.

Rogers, Carl R. "A Theory of Personality." In Millon, ed., *Theories*, 1973.

Rolston, Holmes, III. "Is There an Ecological Ethic?" *Ethics* 85 (Jan. 1975), 93–109.

Schnall, Peter L., and Kern, Rochelle. "Hypertension in American Society: An Introduction to Historical Materialist Epidemiology." In Peter Conrad and Rochelle Kern, eds., *The Sociology of Health and Illness*, pp. 97–121. New York: St. Martins, 1981.

Schrag, Peter. *Mind Control*. New York: Dell, 1978.

Sidel, Victor W., and Sidel, Ruth. *A Healthy State: An International Perspective on the Crisis in United States Medical Care*. New York: Pantheon, 1977.

Silverman, Milton, and Lee, Philip R. *Pills, Profits, and Politics*. Berkeley: University of California Press, 1974.

Skinner, B. F. "What is Psychotic Behavior?" In Millon, ed., *Theories*, 1973, pp. 324–337.

Stark, Evan. "The Epidemic as a Social Event." *International Journal of Health Services* 7, no. 4 (1977), 681–705.

Stellman, Jeanne M., and Daum, Susan M. *Work Is Dangerous to Your Health*. New York: Random House, Vintage Books, 1973.

Stevens, Rosemary. *American Medicine and the Public Interest.*
New Haven: Yale University Press, 1971.

Sullivan, Harry Stack. "The Modified Psychoanalytic Treatment of
Schizophrenia." In Millon, ed., *Theories*, 1973, pp. 217–227.

Szasz, Thomas. *Ideology and Insanity: Essays on the Psychiatric
Dehumanization of Man.* Garden City, N.Y.: Doubleday, Anchor Books, 1970.

————. "Mental Illness as a Metaphor." *Nature* 242 (Mar. 30,
1973), 305–307.

Taylor, Ronald. "Hunger: Knock on Any Door." In Lerza and Jacobson, eds., *Food for People*, 1975, pp. 93–98.

Toulmin, Stephen. "Concepts of Function and Mechanism in Medicine and Medical Science." In Engelhardt and Spiker, eds.,
Evaluation and Explanation, 1975, pp. 51–66.

Ullmann, Leonard P., and Krasner, Leonard. "The Psychological
Model." In Millon, ed., *Theories*, 1973, pp. 338–350.

Versenyi, Laslo. "On Deriving Categorical Imperatives from the
Concept of Action." *Ethics* 86 (July 1976), 265–273.

Vonder Harr, T. A. "Chaining Children with Chemicals." *The Progressive* 39 (Mar. 1975), 13–17.

Weber, Max. *From Max Weber.* Edited and translated by H. H.
Gerth and C. Wright Mills. New York: Oxford University Press,
1958.

Willis, Roy. "Magic and Medicine in Ufipa." In Morley and Wallis,
eds., *Culture and Curing*, 1979, pp. 139–151.

Woods, William. "The Disabled Vet and His $20 Billion Bureau-
cracy." *Rolling Stone*, Feb. 9, 1978.

Zwerdling, Daniel. "The New Pesticide Threat." In Lerza and
Jacobson, eds., *Food for People*, 1975, pp. 311–319.

INDEX

UNIVERSITY PRESS OF NEW ENGLAND publishes books under its own imprint and is the publisher for Brandeis University Press, Brown University Press, University of Connecticut, Dartmouth College, Middlebury College Press, University of New Hampshire, University of Rhode Island, Tufts University, University of Vermont, Wesleyan University Press, and Salzburg Seminar.

Library of Congress Cataloging-in-Publication Data

Wright, Will.
    The social logic of health / Will Wright.
        p.   cm.
    Originally published: New Brunswick, N.J. : Rutgers University Press,
© 1982. With new pref.
    Includes bibliographical references and index.
    ISBN 0–8195–6283–1 (pbk.)
    1. Social medicine.   2. Health.   3. Medicine—Philosophy.   I. Title.
    [DNLM: 1. Philosophy, Medical.   2. Attitude to Health.   W 61
W954s   1982a]
    RA418.W74   1994
    306.4'61—dc20
    DNLM/DLC for Library of Congress   94–34212